Frontiers of Nutrition and Food Security

in Asia, Africa,

and Latin America

Papers and Proceedings

of a Colloquium

Organized by the

Smithsonian Institution

and the International

Life Sciences Institute

North America

Editor and Desktop Publishing Specialist:
Craig A. Reynolds

Manufactured in the United States of
America
99 98 97 96 95 94 93 92 5 4 3 2 1

The paper used in this publication meets
the minimum requirements of the American National Standard for Permanence of
Paper for Printed Library Materials Z39.48-
1984

Volumes in this series are based on annual
colloquia organized at the Smithsonian Institution, in cooperation with the Kraft General Foods Foundation and the Winrock
International Institute for Agricultural Research.

Previously published:

Science, Ethics, and Food, edited by Brian
W. J. Lemay (Smithsonian Institution
Press, 1988).

Completing the Food Chain, edited by
Paula M. Hirschoff and Neil G. Kotler
(Smithsonian Institution Press, 1989).

Sharing Innovation, edited by Neil G. Kotler (Smithsonian Institution Press, 1990).

Library of Congress Cataloging-in-Publica-
tion Data
Frontiers of nutrition and food security in
Asia, Africa, and Latin America / edited by
Neil G. Kotler.
p. cm.
''Papers and proceedings of a colloquium
organized by the Smithsonian Institution.''
Includes bibliographic references.
ISBN 1-56098-145-8 (pbk. : alk. paper)
(Smithsonian)
ISBN 971-22-0022-1 (IRRI)
1. Food supply—Developing countries—
Congresses.
2. Nutrition—Developing countries—Con-
gresses.
I. Kotler, Neil G., 1941–
II. Smithsonian Institution.
HD9018.D442F76   1992
363.8'09172'4—dc20   91-42322

British Library Cataloguing-in-Publication
Data is available

Frontiers of Nutrition and Food Security

Edited by Neil G. Kotler

Published in cooperation with ILSI N.A.

Smithsonian Institution Press

Washington and London

Contents

Foreword

Robert McC. Adams
Secretary, Smithsonian Institution

Green Revolution agricultural science and technology led to greater progress in the past twenty-five years in meeting the food grain needs of the world than had been achieved in any comparable period in history.

Future advances in agriculture, making possible an increase in global food output in the range of 4 percent annually, will be necessary to keep pace with world population growth. Yet increases in the food supply alone will not ensure the long sought after goal of food security, which the World Bank defines as "access by all people at all times to enough food for an active and healthy life."

Stabilizing population growth while increasing the food supply, safeguarding the natural resource base, and accelerating economic growth are, to be sure, the pivotal elements of long-range planning. Of equal importance is the meshing of these macroeconomic forces with the more immediate and near-term challenges of banishing hunger, malnutrition, and disease that affect the survival of hundreds of millions of human beings.

Unfortunately, there are few counterparts in the fields of nutrition and public health to the extraordinary achievements in world agriculture. This is not for lack of research and knowledge. Great advances have been made in assessing the incidence and distribution of undernutrition and in identifying the means of reducing hunger and malnutrition. Much is known about the effects of substandard levels of food energy and micronutrient intake on disease and mortality, cognitive and behavioral dysfunction, reproductive disorders, and human productivity loss. The interaction between malnutrition and infectious disease is well documented. The effectiveness of growth monitoring of infants and children and of food supplementation and fortification interventions is firmly established. Yet harnessing this vast body of knowledge to the exigencies of daily life has not kept pace.

A few statistics tell the story. More than 340 million people in the nations of Africa, Asia, and Latin America are affected by severe undernourishment. Of these, an estimated 140 million children suffer from stunted intellectual and physical capacity. Approximately 60 percent of pregnant women and 50 percent of children below four years of age in these regions suffer from iron-deficiency anemia. Vitamin A deficiency affects an estimated 53 million children in sixteen nations of Africa alone. An estimated two hundred million people, mainly in Asia, suffer from iodine deficiency.

A far broader development agenda is needed to achieve both economic growth and greater equity in the distribution of food and health resources. This would be equivalent to a second-stage transformation emphasizing the behavioral, health, and nutritional sciences and building upon the achievements in agriculture. The focal points would be: the creation of sustainable programs centered on food-based solutions for long-term disease prevention; linkage and coordination of agricultural, economic, nutrition, and health policies; and substantial investment in education and training, and in programs that motivate people to adopt more healthful practices.

In pursuit of solutions, the Smithsonian Institution is honored to have joined with the International Life Sciences Institute-North America in convening the colloquium, "Frontiers of Nutrition and Food Security in Asia, Africa, and Latin America."

Foreword

Alex Malaspina
*President, International Life Sciences Institute-
North America*

The North American branch of the International Life Sciences Institute (ILSI) is pleased to join with the Smithsonian Institution in making available the papers and discussions from the symposium "Frontiers of Nutrition and Food Security in Asia, Africa, and Latin America," along with the deliberations from a follow-up round-table discussion held at ILSI-North America's Washington, D.C., offices. Both events were held in conjunction with the World Food Prize award ceremonies, which took place 17 October 1990.

It is fitting that this book and its predecessor symposium are the product of the first collaboration between ILSI-North America and the Smithsonian Institution. ILSI, a nonprofit scientific organization with seven branches worldwide, is concerned with nutrition, food safety, and environmental issues. It is a nongovernmental organization of the World Health Organization and has specialized consultative status with the Food and Agriculture Organization of the United Nations.

ILSI-North America, formerly known as ILSI-Nutrition Foundation, has a long-standing record of involvement in international nutrition in both developing and developed nations. It serves as secretariat for the International Vitamin A Consultative Group (IVACG), International Nutritional Anemia Consultative Group (INACG), International Nutritional Planners Forum, and International Nutrition Network Exchange. These four programs are managed through a cooperative agreement with the U.S. Agency for International Development.

While these programs and others are doing much to resolve widespread issues of malnutrition and food security, a great deal remains to be done. Toward this end, ILSI-North America is gratified to have had this opportunity to collaborate with the Smithsonian Institution in presenting the symposium and in producing this book. We hope the information in this volume will be read by decision makers and policy analysts everywhere who are concerned with the safety, quality, and availability of the world's food supplies and the nutritional well-being of its inhabitants.

Acknowledgements

This volume contains the papers and proceedings of an international colloquium on food, nutrition, and agriculture that was held at the Smithsonian Institution in Washington, D.C. on 17–18 October 1990.

The colloquium, "Frontiers of Nutrition and Food Security in Asia, Africa, and Latin America," explored research advances in India and China on the malnutrition-infection complex and on the control of micronutrient deficiencies; innovative approaches to nutrition and health policy and planning in Chile and in southern Africa; and successful programs of nutrition education, public health, and behavioral change at the community level. The colloquium papers focused on nutrition and food security issues in nonindustrialized nations of the world, while the panel discussions introduced the perspectives of international research and development.

Colloquium participants reconvened on the morning of 18 October 1991 at the International Life Sciences Institute (ILSI)-North America to discuss new directions for research and policy arising from the ideas generated at the previous day's colloquium. Considerable discussion focused on the ways to strengthen the linkage between agricultural research and development, on the one hand, and nutrition and health, on the other. An edited version of the transcript of the two-hour roundtable discussion is included in this volume.

The 1990 colloquium and published volume represent the fourth in a series of programs examining new directions in agriculture, food policy, and nutritional science. The series has been organized at the Smithsonian Institution in conjunction with the annual award of the World Food Prize, the most prestigious international prize in the fields of agriculture, food policy, and nutrition. The first colloquium, convened in October 1987, generated a book entitled *Science, Ethics, and Food* (Smithsonian Institution Press, 1988). A second colloquium, held in October 1988, resulted in the publication *Completing the Food Chain: Strategies for Combating Hunger and Malnutrition* (Smithsonian Institution Press, 1989). The third colloquium, held in October 1989, generated a volume entitled *Sharing Innovation: Global Perspectives on Food, Agriculture, and Rural Development* (Smithsonian Institution Press, 1990).

The colloquium series, the published volumes, and the awarding of the World Food Prize share a common purpose: to expand knowledge of the applications of agricultural research, food and nutritional science, and of food technologies in feeding the world's population; to bring together leaders from diverse fields to exchange ideas and perspectives on finding solutions to malnutrition and hunger; to examine food issues cross-nationally, especially in the nonindustrialized nations; and to honor individuals who devoted their lives to the goal of generating an ample supply of wholesome food in the world.

This volume is enriched by the inclusion of the remarks of Dr. John S. Niederhauser, who was awarded the 1990 World Food Prize on 17 October in ceremonies held in the Baird Auditorium of the Smithsonian's National Museum of Natural History. Dr. Niederhauser was honored for his successful work in controlling potato late blight disease and for his leadership in building cooperative research and training programs and multinational potato research institutions, all of which have led to the remarkable increase in potato production and consumption throughout the world. Dr. Niederhauser's essay is an expanded version of his remarks upon accepting the World Food Prize.

The 1990 colloquium was jointly developed by Timothy A. Morck of the International Life Sciences Institute-North America and Neil G. Kotler of the Smithsonian's Office of Interdisciplinary Studies (OIS). Cheryl B. LaBerge, Karen Harmon, and Sheri Price of the Smithsonian's Office of Conference Services brought a high degree of professionalism to the support services, in arranging the colloquium events and the travel and lodging of the participants. Carla M. Borden of OIS provided important oversight of the manuscript production.

Several individuals deserve to be cited for their particular contributions to the colloquium and to the published volume. The colloquium program would not have taken place without the participation of eleven distinguished scholars and practitioners who in many cases had traveled considerable distances to take part in the program. Their willingness to share their ideas and experiences made the colloquium a lively and productive event. In addition, their cooperation in working with the editor to clarify and revise their papers, whenever necessary, is very much appreciated.

Dr. Abraham Horwitz was doubly generous in agreeing to serve as a commentator in the colloquium's afternoon session, and in agreeing to write an introduction to the volume. Reflecting an extraordinary career in the fields of nutrition and public health, devoted particularly to his native land of Chile and in his work at the Pan American Health Organization to improving the quality of health and nutrition for peoples throughout Latin America, his experience was of great benefit in helping to shape the colloquium program and the publication.

Dr. Barbara A. Underwood graciously agreed to serve as chairperson in the colloquium's morning session and, at the close of the colloquium, to present a summation of the day's highlights and proceedings. Her summation was superb.

Dr. Robert F. Chandler, Jr., the 1988 World Food Prize laureate and founding director of the International Rice Research Institute (IRRI), shared his unique insights on world agriculture and economic development during the 18 October roundtable discussion, and as he has done in the previous three colloquium programs, he proved to be a highly engaging participant.

Timothy A. Morck of the ILSI-North America chaired the 18 October roundtable discussion with thoughtfulness and sensitivity. Roberta Gutman, publications manager at ILSI-North America, has been continuously helpful in coordinating the publication arrangements with her institution. Vivian B. Morris, a veteran Smithsonian Institution volunteer, performed excellent work in transcribing the tapes of the panel discussions and the colloquium summation.

Recognition is owed to the International Rice Research Institute's support of the publication series. Thomas R. Hargrove, head of communications and information at IRRI, has worked ably with the Smithsonian Institution Press in bringing the published volume to the attention of readers in many parts of the world.

Dr. Craig A. Reynolds, an editor at the Smithsonian Institution Press, deserves a special recognition for his role as copy editor of this volume. His skills in reviewing the text, shaping its form, and in bringing clarity to the text and the illustrations, all contributed to the readability and the quality of the volume.

Two individuals who worked on the 1990 World Food Prize deserve recognition not only in producing a delightful set of events in honoring the 1990 World Food Prize laureate, but also in achieving a smooth transition in prize sponsorship in 1991 from the Kraft General Foods Foundation to the John Ruan Foundation and the The World Food Prize Foundation, both of which are located in Des Moines, Iowa. They are A. S. Clausi, chairman of the Council of Advisors of the World Food Prize, and Edward S. Williams, of the Winrock International Institute for Agricultural Development, which administered the prize in its first four years.

Acknowledgements would not be complete without expressing special appreciation to Dr. Alex Malaspina, president of ILSI-North America, for his keen interest in the colloquium series and for initiating ILSI sponsorship of the 1990 colloquium program and publication. ILSI support was generous and consistent throughout the planning and implementing of the colloquium program. Without Dr. Malaspina's support and that of his institution, neither the colloquium nor this volume would have come into being.

CHAPTER 1

Introduction

Abraham Horwitz
Director Emeritus, Pan American Sanitary Bureau
Pan American Health Organization
Washington, D.C.

The development of technologies, as well as the analysis of experiences in a number of countries, suggests that there are now courses of action, i.e., strategies, that can be applied to alleviate nutrition problems and improve the human condition, without having to wait for the longer process of redressing social inequities. Perhaps more important, there is a consensus that the intersectoral plans and actions that characterized thinking in the 1960s and 1970s are not a prerequisite for progress. This conclusion does not argue against synergistic effects of multiple approaches. Rather, it does argue that the complex planning process designed earlier, which by its very complexity convinced many planners that nothing really could be accomplished within the practical world, itself is not essential.

Sector-Based Interventions

As has been stated, the fact that nutrition problems have multiple causes does not mean that all causes have to be addressed at the same time. It follows that a better approach is to select and implement validated sectoral actions that are cost-effective.

Nutrition as an outcome has become the basis for policy and program formulation and implementation. It reflects the results of well-proven interventions—or clusters of them—that can reduce progressively undernutrition and malnutrition. Although sector-based, many of these interventions benefit from combined effects when concurrently applied. On the other hand, single-sector interventions can have positive outcomes and should not, therefore, be discarded. There is evidence that

1

actions in health, education, agriculture, food supplementation, income generation or transfer, and others, can have a significant impact in improving food consumption and utilization and, thus, the nutritional status of people.

Five clusters of interventions have been identified that deal directly with highly frequent nutrition problems or diet-associated diseases occurring in the developing world. In terms of decisions, they focus more on individuals and communities than on the national level. They are:

1. household food security;
2. the control of the malnutrition-infection complex;
3. caring capacity, behavior, and the use of available resources by mothers;
4. the control of micronutrient deficiencies;
5. diet and prevention of chronic diseases.

This distribution of nutritional issues and clustering of potential solutions is for operational purposes. It is rooted in solid scientific bases and responds to the most prevalent and critical health and nutrition problems in Asia, Africa, and Latin America. On the other hand, it emphasizes the fundamental contribution of women to secure the nutritional status of all family members. Governments, of course, may select among these or other issues and interventions.

Contemporary Approaches

The colloquium "Frontiers of Nutrition and Food Security in Asia, Africa, and Latin America" reflects, in my view, the best contemporary approaches to nutrition policy and planning, and some of the major interventions that we have just enunciated. From this angle, the colloquium has made an important contribution. However, it should have further effects, because it dealt with nutritional problems prevalent in the developing world. In his elegant and concise presentation, Smithsonian Secretary Robert McC. Adams refers to the large numbers of mothers and children in the three regions who suffer from chronic undernutrition and micronutrient deficiencies. In analyzing these conditions, the colloquium showed the effective technologies in use that can be replicated in different ecological settings, and that can be made sustainable by communities and governments, thus advancing food security. The colloquium papers add to the literature on successful nutrition programs, carefully evaluated, in the world. Although the road ahead may be long, as expressed by the numbers of the undernourished and malnourished, we have now clear pathways leading to the solution of their problem. Science, therefore, has provided—and continues to provide—validated knowledge and technologies to progressively improve the nutritional status of people who live in poverty and deprivation. Governments and the international nutrition community of technical and financial cooperation have the responsibility to accelerate this process. Again, the colloquium has added valuable experiences.

Micronutrient Deficiencies

Two of the papers dealt with prevalent micronutrient deficiencies in the developing world, vitamin A and iron. Dr. V. Rahmathullah provided concrete evidence that a small dose of vitamin A, equivalent to the recommended daily intake, reduced by 54 percent mortality rates of preschool children that resulted from acute infections. In contrast to this dramatic effect on mortality, vitamin A supplementation did not influence morbidity rates, a disparity the author attributes to "the overwhelming synergistic effect in the poverty-stricken areas we studied in India of a contaminated environment and poor personal sanitary habits."

Dr. Rahmathullah's study is certainly in the frontiers of nutrition and food security, not only because of its results but also because of its implications for the developing world. Nutritional blindness can be prevented and death due to certain acute infections reduced in preschool children, by increasing the regular consumption of carotene B-rich food, available in practically all countries. If these products are not accessible, then vitamin A supplementation and fortification should be considered. At the same time, environmental stresses reflected in infections, behaviors that induce disease, lack of water, basic sanitation and personal hygiene, illiteracy, and other causes, should be controlled at the community level, thus increasing the impact of vitamin A.

Because it focuses on the most populous country in the world, The People's Republic of China, and also because it examines the most prevalent micronutrient deficiency, namely, iron deficiency, the article by Dr. Liu Dong-sheng is significant to all countries. Dr. Liu summarizes a series of studies on the prevalence of iron-deficiency anemia in preschool children and in pregnant mothers. Rates are high, and the problem can be prevented or controlled because causes are known and effective technologies are available. She refers particularly to iron supplementation and iron fortification, the latter on the basis of a series of food staples common in China. However, Dr. Liu considers nutrition education in terms of human resources development as perhaps the most important approach for the eradication of iron deficiency—an important message for all countries of the world.

National and Regional Policy

After examining specific micronutrient deficiencies, the colloquium analyzed chronic undernutrition and malnutrition in a single country as a whole, in Chile. Dr. Fernando Monckeberg presented a successful national experience, demonstrating why and how in Chile sustained policies and interventions, over thirty years, have substantially reduced mortality, morbidity, and malnutrition and increased birth weight and life expectancy to levels similar to those of a number of industrialized societies. This progress has occurred, according to Dr. Monckeberg, in spite

3

of several economic crises, intermittent economic stagnation, and political upheavals.

Continuity in decisions, investments, and actions to transfer national income to the people through social services, health, and nutrition explains the success in Chile and serves, among others, as a lesson for developing countries. This approach could be adapted to the political, economic, cultural, and environmental conditions of other nations that face similar health and nutrition problems. In fact, during the same three decades, several countries in the Americas also have reached comparable levels of progress. Others, in the same or different regions, could follow through.

Africa shows a need for a continuous process of capacity building and institutional development in order to achieve the critical mass of human resources and skills that is essential to undertake effective food security and nutrition programs. Ms. Maribe presents a model developed in the East, Central, and Southern African countries known as ECSA Food/Nutrition Cooperation and the mechanisms for coordinating activities among the countries. This model includes the institutions available in the region for formal and in-service training. It is suggested that a similar approach could be developed in other regions of Africa. The nutrition problems examined are typical of developing societies, and the programs prepared, according to Ms. Maribe, cannot be successfully developed "unless basic requirements regarding human and institutional needs are met."

In a region with such a high incidence of undernutrition and of the malnutrition-infection complex—besides a famine crisis in some countries—the colloquium is proposing a clear approach towards the solution of these problems in the medium and long term.

Social Marketing and Behavior Modification

Experience has shown an urgent need for large numbers of people to change their behavior in order to prevent disease and to promote health. They face increasing risks, particularly where poverty, malnutrition, and deprivation prevail; and these risks occur in developed and developing societies alike in relation to different conditions. Changing behavior requires an iterative process, culture-specific, based on messages carefully designed, and addressed to target populations. Behavioral change also requires communication methodologies rooted in the knowledge of biological and social sciences. In comparison to certain addictions, behavioral change related to acute infections and malnutrition can be brought about in a relatively short period of time. Then, it becomes sustainable and transferable, because it depends on the new knowledge, attitudes, and practices of the people.

Dr. Eduardo L. Roberto has made an important contribution with his chapter. He considers social marketing as a management practice, a discipline of imple-

4

mentation. Roberto's approach is pragmatic. Other practitioners of the art believe that it is "a strategy for translating scientific findings about health and nutrition into education and action programs adopted from methodologies of commercial marketing."[1] Still others think that the old discipline of health and nutrition education, modernized with the concepts and methodologies of the biological and social sciences, could lead to the expected results, namely, changing people's behavior to avert death, prevent disease, and promote health. They see no need for the principles and tools of commercial marketing. Further experiences will be useful to determine which of these approaches is most cost-effective to reach this essential goal.

The presentation of the papers, the comments of the discussants, and the dialogue with the audience, all contributed to bringing clarity to the concepts and results, identifying research issues, and showing what must be done to conquer the frontiers of nutrition and food security in Asia, Africa, and Latin America. The readers of this volume of colloquium papers and proceedings, who were not privileged to attend the sessions, will certainly benefit from the wealth of insight and experience that it contains.

Notes

1.   Richard R. Manoff, *Social Marketing: A New Imperative for Public Health* (Westport, Conn.: Prager and Greenwood Publishers, 1985), 36.

CHAPTER 2

Effects of Frequent, Low-Dose Vitamin A Intake on Child Survival: Implications for Community-Based Programs

V. Rahmathullah
Director, Child Development Unit
Aravind Children's Hospital
Madurai, India

Twenty to forty million children worldwide are estimated at any one time to be suffering from at least mild vitamin A deficiency. The Subcommittee on Nutrition of the United Nations has estimated that nearly half of those affected reside in India.[1] The majority of the remaining afflicted children live in parts of Southeast Asia and of Africa. That severe deficiency leads to blindness is well known, but the fact that subclinical deficiency also has consequences has only recently been recognized.

The potential worldwide implications of subclinical vitamin A deficiency for child health and survival were suggested in a series of studies from Indonesia in the mid-1980s. These studies reported a marked increase in the risk of diarrheal and respiratory morbidity[2] and risk of mortality associated with these symptoms.[3] Providing a large dose of vitamin A to Indonesian children was reported to have reduced mortality by at least 34 percent.[4] A similar intervention among children in Thailand reportedly reduced morbidity as well.[5] An earlier community-based study in Thailand that had distributed vitamin A-fortified rice, however, demonstrated no health effects,[6] whereas vitamin A-fortified monosodium glutamate, marketed in Indonesia, reduced risk of mortality, decreased anemia, and stimulated growth as well.[7] In India one study demonstrated that risk was elevated for respiratory morbidity but, in contrast to the Indonesia findings, risk was not elevated for diarrhea in mildly xerophthalmic children (i.e., children suffering from vitamin A deficiency and exhibiting clinical signs such as night blindness, Bitot spots, or scars).[8] In the Indonesian study children with vitamin A deficiency were at risk of getting both diarrhea and respiratory infection. Because of these varied results and, in some cases, with questions about design of the early studies,[9] planners and policy makers in areas with endemic vitamin A deficiency have been uncertain about how to set priorities for child survival programs, all of which have to compete for limited resources. Even if the public health consequences of vitamin A deficiency are firmly delineated, local communities and national planners alike face the problem of selecting which interventions (e.g., supplementation with low- or high-dose vitamin A or through food sources) best suit their needs and are affordable and sustainable.[10]

To answer some of the scientific and feasibility questions in India, as well as in other countries where the dietary intake of vitamin A by young children is very inadequate, and at the same time to provide guidance for future program planning, we conducted a randomized, controlled, masked clinical trial among over 15,400 preschool-aged children. We used a small dose of vitamin A, equivalent to the recommended daily intake, but administered it weekly (i.e., 8.7 micro mole, or 8,333 International Units [IU]). This amount was given as a liquid vitamin A supplement for the purposes of the control needed in a research study involving such a large number of children. However, it is an amount achievable through foods that could compose the diet of weanling and preschool-aged children almost anywhere in the world.

Study Design and Implementation

The study was carried out in three drought-prone, economically, and environmentally deprived Panchayat Unions (i.e., group of villages forming a political unit) of Trichi District in Tamil Nadu in southern India. The populations in the areas chosen had been underserved by child-care programs, including a national program in which a large-dose supplement of vitamin A is administered every six months Only 1 percent of the children under five years had participated in this program.

The study was conducted with the participation and approval of community leaders and workers, wherever feasible. Local political and professional leaders assisted with prestudy publicity and cooperated by nominating individuals to staff up the project. Enumerators and local workers were recruited from these lists after training and performance evaluations. They mapped the areas and obtained demographic information from all households. This research included a five-year survey involving mothers with children under the age of five years who had died. An external medical team that included social workers and local volunteers conducted a baseline ocular and medical examination, obtained anthropometric measurements, and elicited a morbidity history. The ocular examination was repeated at midterm, and the entire examination protocol was repeated at the end of the study. In addition, a random sample of 2 percent of the children contributed a finger prick blood sample so that researchers could determine their vitamin A levels. Also, for

Table 2-1

Baseline Characteristics of the Study Population

	(%)		(%)
Sex		**Serum Retinol** (mmol/l)	
Males	52	≤ .35	21.4
Females	48	.35–.70	16.1
Age[1] (months)		.701–1.05	16.4
≤ 5	1.8	>1.05	46.1
6–11	7.1	**Nutritional Status**[2]	
12–23	20.0	Stunted	31
24–35	21.0	Wasted	23
36–47	22.1	Stunted and	
48–60	22.4	Wasted	18
61–71	5.4	Normal	25
Xerophthalmia Status		Unknown	3
Night blindness	3.7		
Bitot's spots	7.2		
Corneal in-			
volvement	0.05		
Scars	0.07		

Source: Data is the author's. Dr. V. Rahmathullah was chief investigator of a Ford Foundation–funded project exploring the effects of vitamin A on morbidity and mortality in preschool children in South India.

Notes: N = 15,419.

[1] Age at start of intervention.

[2] As determined using the CDC Anthropometric Software Package (CASP), version 3.

STUNTED = height/age < (mean - 2 standard deviations [SD]) and weight/height ≥ (mean - 2SD). Stunting results from prolonged, inadequate food intake. A stunted child is shorter than normal.

WASTED = height/age ≥ (mean - 2SD) and weight/height < (mean - 2SD). Wasting results when a person consumes too few calories to maintain a weight proportionate to his or her height. Wasting is synonymous with acute undernutrition.

STUNTED AND WASTED = height/age < (mean - 2SD) and weight/height < (mean - 2SD). Stunted and wasted indicate a prolonged and acute condition of inadequate dietary intake.

NORMAL = height/age ≥ (mean - 2SD) and weight/height ≥ (mean - 2 SD).

each of these children a dietary history was taken that probed the frequency of intake of locally available vitamin A-rich foods. All the children who at any time exhibited symptoms of xerophthalmia, including night blindness, were given a large-dose supplement of vitamin A and were kept in their randomized treatment group for observation.

After enumeration, all children, six to sixty months of age, were grouped into clusters composed of fifty to one hundred children, and the clusters were randomly assigned to receive on a weekly basis either a supplement containing vitamins A and E (i.e., the treatment group), or vitamin E alone (i.e., the control group). A trained community health volunteer (CHV) was put in charge of the weekly dispensing of the appropriate color-coded vitamin supplement to each child in her or his cluster. The CHV also obtained a week-long history of the children's morbidity symptoms, with special attention given to diarrhea and to respiratory diseases.

Table 2-2

Weekly Coverage of Study Children and Minimum Vitamin A Received According to Coverage

Doses Missed	Cumulative Coverage Children (%) (N = 15,419)	Minimum Dose Received Vitamin A (international units, in thousands)
0	41.8	433
1–5	80.5	392
6–10	87.4	350
11–15	90.6	308
16–20	92.6	267
21–26	94.3	217
27–31	95.0	175

Source: Data is the author's.

The baseline characteristics of the study population, provided in Table 2-1, were not different for the two treatment groups. The results revealed a high prevalence of protein-energy undernutrition (72 percent) and of clinical (11 percent) and biochemical (21 percent) vitamin A deficiency. Biochemical data, in fact, suggested that one-third to one-half of the children had inadequate vitamin A levels (i.e., less than 0.70 or 1.05 micro mole per liter).

Results

Coverage
Distribution of the supplement began uniformly on the same date and continued for fifty-two weeks. Through the implementation of a hierarchical personnel and

data management supervision and review scheme, the study achieved strict control over the completeness and accuracy of the data collected. Coverage by CHVs exceeded 90 percent for most weeks, the lowest weekly coverage being 88 percent of the children contacted. Forty-two percent of the children received every dose, which was equivalent to 433,000 IU (Table 2-2). This amount is similar to what they would have received if they had been part of the six-month, large-dose, national program of India, which is implemented through the health system.

Mortality

Of 125 deaths that occurred (i.e., a mortality rate of 8.1 per 1000), 117 were non-accidental and were associated with the symptoms reported in Table 2-3. As can be seen, deaths occurred in association with symptoms indicative of a concurrent infection. Table 2-4 shows the relative risk of death by age and treatment group. The age-adjusted overall risk was reduced by 54 percent for those who received the small weekly dose of vitamin A, as compared with the control group. All ages in the treated group benefitted, but the protective effect was most pronounced in those children under one year of age (risk reduction of 72 percent) and in the children one to three years of age. Figure 2-1 shows the cumulative deaths that occurred by treatment group. Obviously, the continuous supply of a small weekly dose of vitamin A began to have its protective effect almost immediately. These results concur with the findings reported from the supplementation studies among Indonesian children.

Table 2-3

Symptoms Associated with Death

Symptom	Deaths (No.)	Symptom	Deaths (No.)
Accidents	8	Measles	19
Convulsions	15	Polio	2
Diarrhea	49	Respiratory	
Encephalitis	5	disorders	5
Fever	6	Tetanus, mumps,	5
Intestinal ob-		cirrhosis, ne-	
structions	3	phritis	5
Jaundice	4		
Malnutrition	4		
		Total	125

Source: Data is the author's.

10

As shown in Table 2-5, the protective effect of the consistent provision of vitamin A was striking for those children suffering from chronic undernutrition or stunting (i.e., those who are smaller in height and weight as a result of a prolonged-state of inadequate food intake). Their risk of fatality was nearly eight times less than was the case for normally nourished children and six times less than for the acutely undernourished, or wasted, children (i.e., those whose inadequate food consumption over limited periods has resulted in weight loss). Stunting, further-more, is that anthropometric measurement most closely associated with poverty conditions in households, including food inaccessibility and insecurity.[11]

Morbidity

In contrast to the dramatic effect on risk of dying, low-dose vitamin A supplemen-tation did not dramatically affect the incidence, duration of an episode, or severity (i.e., as reflected by the total number of days ill) of either diarrhea (defined as four or more loose or watery stools in a day) or of respiratory illnesses (defined either as mild upper respiratory [URI] or more severe lower respiratory [LRI] symptoms lasting at least three days). During the one-year period of observation, children suffered from nearly six episodes of diarrhea of an average four days duration per episode, regardless of their baseline nutritional status. Over half of the children had at least one episode of URI and 4 percent of them had at least one episode of LRI. As with diarrhea, the baseline nutritional status was unrelated to incidence, duration of an episode, or severity of respiratory illnesses.

Our inability to demonstrate an influence of vitamin A treatment or of base-line nutritional status on diarrhea or respiratory morbidity in the Indian children contrasts with the reports of protective effects in observational studies in Indonesia and intervention studies in Thailand. This disparity in findings likely reflects the overwhelming synergistic effect in the poverty-stricken areas we studied in India of a contaminated environment and poor personal sanitary habits.

Growth

The vitamin A supplementation studies conducted in Indonesia demonstrated im-proved linear or ponderal growth during a one year observation period. Our study, however, did not detect growth related to treatment. The reason for the lack of growth in our study may lie in the pervasive protein-energy malnutrition (PEM) in the Indian population that appears to be of greater severity than in Indonesia[12] and may have been more growth-limiting than vitamin A deficiency. Also, it is well-documented that frequent diarrheal infections are associated with growth decelera-tion,[13] and the high incidence of diarrhea in our study was not altered by treatment.

We observed an interesting growth phenomenon that was unrelated to vitamin A treatment. Children who were stunted at the beginning of the study showed the greatest annualized increment in linear growth, greater than those children who

Table 2-4

Mortality by Age and Treatment Group

Age (months)	Treatment Group	Children (no.)	Deaths	Prevalence Rate	Relative Risk[1]	Confidence Interval (95%)
0–11	control	678	14	0.021	0.28*	(0.09, 0.85)
	treated	689	4	0.006		
12–35	control	3,185	52	0.016	0.46**	(0.26, 0.81)
	treated	3,179	24	0.008		
≥36	control	3,792	14	0.004	0.63	(0.26, 1.50)
	treated	3,896	9	0.002		
Total	control	7,655	80	0.010	0.46**	(0.29, 0.71)
	treated	7,764	37	0.005		
Total	age-adjusted				0.46**	(0.30, 0.71)

Source: Data is the author's.

Notes: [1] represents a measure of the risk of having the condition when the treated group is compared with the control group.
* Significant at $p = 0.05$.
** Significant at both $p = 0.05$ and $p = 0.01$.

Figure 2-1

Weekly Totals of Cumulative Deaths for Both Control and Vitamin A–treated Groups of Preschool Children, Over the Fifty-two Weeks of the Study

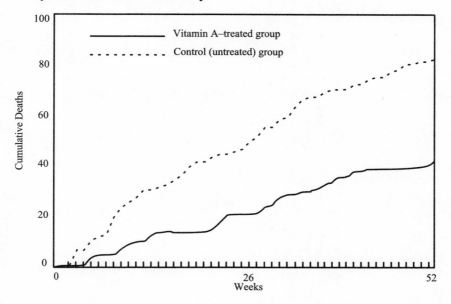

entered the study with normal height for age, and considerably greater than those who entered the study acutely underweight for their age. As already mentioned, stunting is an anthropometric surrogate for several household, poverty-related conditions. Perhaps the explanation for this greater response in catch-up growth among children presumably from the most chronically deprived households is the contact effect. Merely being systematically visited and questioned by a local worker who may not even be trained to administer health care directly can, as suggested by Dr. Gopalan,[14] lead to improvements in food intake that can alter some of those poverty-related conditions that retard child development.

Implications of This Study

The study I have just reviewed demonstrated that there can be a striking effect on child survival of modestly improving the level of vitamin A intake in chronically undernourished, vitamin A-depleted children. This potentially can be achieved by increasing their consumption of vitamin A-rich food during the early years of life,

Table 2-5

Mortality by Nutritional Status

Status[1]	Treatment Group	Children (no.)	Deaths (no.)	Prevalence Rate	Relative Risk [2]	Confidence Interval (95%)
Stunted	control	2,385	27	.011	0.11*	(0.03, 0.36)
	treated	2,418	3	.001		
Wasted	control	1,806	14	.008	0.72	(0.30, 1.72)
	treated	1,798	10	.006		
Stunted and wasted	control	1,373	22	.016	0.65	(0.30, 1.41)
	treated	1,340	14	.010		
Normal	control	1,890	11	.006	0.80	(0.32, 2.00)
	treated	1,940	9	.005		

Source: Data is the author's.

Notes: [1] As determined using the CDC Anthropometric Software Package (CASP), version 3. STUNTED = height/age ≥ (mean - 2 standard deviations [SD]) and weight/height ≥ (mean - 2SD); WASTED = height/age ≥ (mean - 2SD) and weight/height (mean - 2SD); STUNTED AND WASTED = height/age < (mean - 2SD) and weight/height < (mean - 2SD); NORMAL = height/age ≥ (mean - 2SD) and weight/height ≥ (mean - 2 SD).
[2] Treated versus control.
* Significant at $p = 0.01$.

or, where accessibility to food is not possible for economic or ecologic reasons, through a community-based, supplement-delivery infrastructure that uses a safe level of supplemental vitamin A. Of equal importance, the study also demonstrated that it will take additional action at the community and household level to control childhood illnesses perpetuated by a contaminated environment and so closely linked to deprivation that constantly challenges and assaults the physiological defense systems of young children. This would include programs that address issues of immunization, environmental sanitation, personal hygiene, access to health care, literacy, traditional child-care practices, and social isolation.

Application for Indian Communities

For India, I would summarize the programmatic implications of our study as follows:

1.   It is imperative to consistently provide the recommended dietary allowance (RDA) to preschool-aged children in areas with a high prevalence of vitamin A deficiency and undernutrition in order to substantially enhance child survival. Locally available natural food sources could provide the level of vitamin A required in most situations;

2.   Maximum survival effects in such areas are most likely to be achieved by targeting programs to the younger age groups, including their mothers and/or caretakers, and to those children who are chronically undernourished, i.e., stunted;

3.   Policies and programs that relieve conditions contributing to stunting (e.g., improving diet, increasing social contacts, and improving socioeconomic conditions) will decrease vitamin A deficiency-related mortality.

The challenge is applying this knowledge gained from a research project in practical programs to relieve the vitamin A deficiency that exists in the various states of India. Rates of vitamin A deficiency vary considerably across the regions. Early surveys indicated that a range of five to fifteen percent of children have clinical signs of deficiency. We found 11 percent with clinical eye signs (i.e., night blindness, Bitot spots, or scars) in our study. One report of a countrywide survey in 1974 indicated that on average 7 percent of all preschool-aged children exhibit such clinical symptoms.[15] Although recently conducted surveys show a declining trend, in many states the prevalence of clinical signs continues to exceed World Health Organization criteria for a public health problem. The number of children in India who are subclinically deficient far exceeds the number with clinically evident deficiency (i.e., up to half of the children in our study area). As we have shown, these children are at high risk of not surviving an infection. Applying our results to the national situation in India should lead to an urgent call for effective vitamin A deficiency control programs as a part of child survival strategies.

15

Current Micronutrient Programs

Current policy in India is to give a large dose of vitamin A at six-month intervals to all children one to five years of age, administered by means of the Primary Health Care (PHC) system. However, only fifteen million children of the eighty million eligible in India are currently receiving the vitamin treatment through this program.[16] It is obvious that India will not solve its vitamin A deficiency problem unless greater efficiency in distribution is achieved.

In India, the PHC system has failed to provide comprehensive health care. One reason for this is the lack of community involvement and the widely held view that the health care system is a bureaucratic governmental operation accessible only as a last recourse.[17] Medical officers in the system lack credibility because they are often newly graduated and are frequently transferred between posts so they do not develop community trust. This psychological distance dividing providers and beneficiaries in the current system can only be bridged by radical qualitative changes in the health/nutrition/welfare operations at the village level.

Some countries have attempted to decrease vitamin A deficiency by fortifying foods. In India, some dairy and tinned milk products (formula milk powder) and vanaspati (margarine), commercially available on the Indian market, are fortified with vitamin A. However, these are too expensive for those most in need of the vitamin. None of the cereals that are the primary dietary component of the poor have production and distribution attributes necessary to become a viable fortification vehicle. Therefore, in India, fortification of an inexpensive food commonly consumed by young children does not seem to be a practical solution to vitamin A deficiency.

Fortunately, India has available the natural foods that potentially can alleviate the problem of vitamin A deficiency. There also exists the necessary information to facilitate the planning of locally appropriate programs. Because of the productive investigations over many years emanating from the National Institute of Nutrition in Hyderabad and from other Indian food and nutrition research units, the vitamin A and carotenoid content of most widely available Indian foods is known.[18] The mean intake of vitamin A in all Indian states and the degree to which it is inadequate also is known, including the pattern of consumption of green leafy vegetables and other foods in the diets of preschool-aged children. Thus, the information and resources are available for establishing food-based vitamin A control programs that are adapted to area-specific community infrastructures and that are accompanied by the dissemination of educational materials to facilitate consumption by young children.

Potential Delivery Systems

The Integrated Child Development Service (ICDS) is one existing program in India that is being evaluated as a potential delivery system for integrated control of

16

vitamin A deficiency. Two-thirds of the country is covered by the program. Each ICDS center serves approximately one thousand children; children up to five years of age are eligible for the program. Those under three can utilize the centers for health care services, but in practice, only children three to five years of age attend the centers and receive the food as well. Each center is managed by a local woman, known as an *Anganwadi* worker, who is primarily responsible for preschool education and who fills a supporting role in health care. Currently, a health worker can use ICDS for the periodic distribution of high-dose vitamin A supplements. Recent evaluations suggest that coverage of children with vitamin A supplement has improved and, in addition, this integrated system has enhanced the utilization of related health services. The improvement is believed to be related to the empowerment of the Anganwadi worker, who is being used increasingly to deliver preventive health services, and to her close identification with the community.

Yet the vitamin A coverage by the health service still remains inadequate. Based on our study, it is my suggestion that the Anganwadi worker be given a solution of vitamin A at a lower dosage level, e.g., a seven-day multiple of the RDA, which she can control and safely dispense. In principle the food provided in the midday meal at the ICDS centers, which serve the three- to five-year-old children, should contain an adequate quantity of vitamin A to meet the RDA, but often the levels are inadequate. The Anganwadi worker could use the low-dose vitamin A supplement to provide a weekly dose of the vitamin (or at some other frequent, safe schedule) to all children in the program regardless of age or, where vitamin A-rich foods for the three- to five-year-old children is adequate, target the vitamin A supplement to children, six months to three years.

In India, the Tamil Nadu Integrated Nutrition Program (TNINP) has been developed to serve women and severely undernourished children (i.e., those with third degree malnutrition) under three years of age. In this program there is one village health worker for every one thousand people, as well as a community nutrition worker for every five TNINP centers. Previously, the concentrated vitamin A supplement used in the national program was given to the TNINP worker for dispensing, and coverage was said to be quite high. However, because of safety concerns, health workers again have taken over the distribution of vitamin A through the TNINP centers, and as a consequence coverage has declined. Experience has shown that the best coverage in the distribution of vitamin A supplements is achieved outside of the national health care system. To turn the program over to other organizational structures, however, requires the availability of a supplement with a safe dosage level so that it does not require strict control over the frequency of distribution.

Another possible direction for improving the coverage of vitamin A supplementation is to integrate delivery with the existing universal immunization program. This program in India is rapidly improving its outreach and it could provide the means for delivery of supplemental vitamin A. This would involve a prophylactic supplement given to children under three years of age to help them build their body reserves in anticipation of an inadequate diet during weaning and early childhood. Such an intervention would safeguard the children until they achieve an age at which they would be reached by other nutrition programs such as ICDS.

Education

Control of vitamin A deficiency will be achieved not only by making the vitamin accessible through food or supplements but also by ensuring its full utilization by the targeted group. The community must understand the importance of the vitamin to family health and child survival, then recognize a need for it, and finally feel empowered to fulfill its need, either by altering family and child diets or by utilizing services that provide the vitamin. Such community action presupposes an educational campaign to raise public awareness of the problems and the means to find the solutions.

Among the people who are in most need of such education are illiterate mothers and young girls. Among these target groups experience has shown that the most powerful means of changing behavior is oral communication. Video is emerging as an effective tool in health education, but this technology is not yet within reach of the majority of rural communities. One-on-one education by means of nonprofessional village women's groups can be an effective medium as long as the messages communicated accurately reflect local circumstances, such as the availability of vitamin A-rich foods and the importance of child feeding practices. Thus, health and nutrition education programs should be cognizant of any literacy and communication problems among the target groups selected for intervention. Where functional literacy classes are being conducted, health and nutrition education should be incorporated as a vital part of the process.

Agricultural Interventions

The agricultural system must become involved in addressing the vitamin A deficiency problem at the community level. Assistance is required to increase the availability of vitamin A-rich foods in rural markets and to promote and support home gardening, wherever feasible.

Our market survey data indicates that the few vitamin A-rich foods available in rural markets are more costly than in urban markets. This obstacle can be overcome if the agricultural department encourages the growing of vitamin A-rich foods in small household plots and assures appropriate distribution so that the market demands of the urban population, as well as of the rural population, are met with products at affordable prices. To date, agriculturalists have been overly occupied with cereal production at the expense of vegetable cultivation. However, small farmers who cannot economically cultivate major cereal crops can be encouraged to transfer production to vitamin A-rich foods, such as vegetables and fruits, e.g., papaya, so long as they are assured that their enterprise will lead to a successful economic outcome.

Limited attempts have been made by the Horticultural Department of the Ministry of Agriculture to promote home gardening in a few major towns in India. Seeds, fertilizers, pesticides, and technical expertise have been provided to housewives to grow vegetables at home and to sell excess produce to the horticultural department through a vegetable cooperative store. This has had two effects: 1) to provide an income for the housewife; and 2) to regulate the market price of vegetables. If this scheme could be extended to rural areas, there is a tremendous potential in making vegetables and fruits (including those rich in vitamin A) available at affordable prices for the rural population as well as generating family income for those who participate as producers. Early efforts to encourage home gardening through various sponsored projects have not been successful except in the cases in which technical advice, seeds, fertilizer, and other supportive services have been provided directly by agriculturalists.

Recommendations for India

For effective control of the problem of vitamin A deficiency in India, current program structures must be expanded, and community-level participation strengthened. One possibility is to mobilize a broad-gauged popular or consumer movement for health and nutrition with the government providing the necessary logistical, technical, and financial support. The following recommendations are made for child survival strategies in a vast country such as India, where it is unlikely that any single method of distribution of vitamin A can be effective:

1. In both the ICDS and TNINP programs workers should be given the responsibility for vitamin A distribution at safe dosage levels. The feeding programs of both organizations should contain adequate vitamin A-rich foods to meet the RDA;

2. The TNINP nutritional supplementation program that now caters only to children under the age of three who suffer from third degree malnutrition should be expanded to include those at the stage when growth starts to falter, and the program should provide vitamin A in the form of food and nutritional supplements;

3. At all ICDS centers the distribution of vitamin A should be through the Anganwadi workers, and the supplement should be made available at safe dosage levels;

4. In areas where ICDS or other nutrition programs do not currently exist, the national PHC system should institute a program of providing low-dosage vitamin A supplements that can be integrated into the ongoing immunization program;

5. Health education programs should aim to achieve behavioral changes and not only be an exercise in information giving;

6. Child development leaders should identify region- and area-specific vita-

min A-rich foods, create imaginative ideas for their preparation that are culturally acceptable in child feeding, and arrange for the production and availability of these foods;

7.   Traditional diets should be reviewed to determine how their vitamin A content might be enhanced through better use of locally available food sources;

8.   Finally, but very importantly, the agricultural community must be involved in the promotion and cultivation, at the local and household level, of vitamin A-rich foods, including the creation of home gardens and cooperative-based production and distribution centers.

Notes

1.   *First Report on the World Nutrition Situation, Administrative Committee on Coordination, Subcommittee on Nutrition,* (New York: United Nations, 1987), 36.

2.   A. Sommer, J. Katz, and I. Tarwotjo, "Increased Risk of Respiratory Disease and Diarrhea in Children with Preexisting Mild Vitamin A Deficiency," *American Journal of Clinical Nutrition* 40 (1984):1090–95.

3.   A. Sommer et al., "Increased Morality in Children with Mild Vitamin A Deficiency", *Lancet* ii (1983):585–88.

4.   A. Sommer et al., "Impact of Vitamin A Supplementation on Childhood Mortality. A Randomized Controlled Community Trial," *Lancet* i (1986):1169–73.

5.   M. W. Bloem et al., "Mild Vitamin A Deficiency and Risk of Respiratory tract Diseases and Diarrhea in Preschool and School Children in Northeastern Thailand," *American Journal of Epidemiology* 131 (1990):332–39.

6.   S. N. Gershoff et al., "Nutrition Studies in Thailand, II. Effects of Fortification of Rice with Lysine, Threonine, Thiamin, Riboflavin, Vitamin A, and Iron on Preschool Children," *American Journal of Clinical Nutrition* 30 (1977):118.

7.   D. Permeisih Muhilal et al., "Vitamin A-fortified Monosodium Glutamate and Health, Growth, and Survival of Children: A Controlled Field Trial," *American Journal of Clinical Nutrition* 48 (1988):1271–76.

8.   R. Milton, V. Reddy, and A. N. Naidu, "Mild Vitamin A Deficiency and Childhood Morbidity—An Indian Experience," *American Journal of Clinical Nutrition* 46 (1987):827–29.

9.   National Research Council, *Vitamin A Supplementation: Methodologies for Field Trials,* (Washington, D.C.: National Academy Press, 1987).

10.   B. A. Underwood, "Vitamin A Prophylaxis Programs in Developing Countries: Past Experiences and Future Prospects," *Nutrition Reviews* 48 (1990):265–74.

11.   R. Martorell and T. J. Ho, "Malnutrition, Morbidity and Mortality," *Population and Development Review* (Supplement to v. 10, 1984):49–68.

12.   K. P. West, Jr. et al., "Vitamin A Supplementation and Growth: A Randomized Community Trial," *American Journal of Clinical Nutrition* 48 (1988):1257–64. See also Note 7.

13.   C. K. Lutter et al., "Nutritional Supplementation: Effects on Child Stunting because of Diarrhea," *American Journal of Clinical Nutrition* 50 (1989):1–8.

14.   C. Gopalan, "Vitamin A and Child Mortality," *Bulletin of the Nutrition Foundation of India* 11 (1990):1–3.

15.   K. Vijayaraghavan et al., "A Simple Method to Evaluate the Massive Dose Vitamin A Prophylaxis Program in Preschool Children," *American Journal of Clinical Nutrition* 45 (1987):970–76.

16.   K. Vijayaraghavan, "Country Reports: India," In: *Proceedings of the National Sympo-*

sium and XIII IVACG Meeting, Kathmandu, Nepal, November 5–10, 1989, (Washington, D.C.: International Life Sciences Institute-Nutrition Foundation, 1990), 36.

17. C. Gopalan and S. Kaur, *Women and Nutrition in India*, Nutrition Foundation of India, Special Publication Series 5:12.

18. C. Gopalan et al., *Diet Atlas of India* (Hyderabad, India: National Institute of Nutrition and Indian Council of Medical Research, 1969).

CHAPTER 3

Strategies to Combat Iron-Deficiency Anemia in China

Liu Dong-sheng
Professor, Institute of Nutrition and Food Hygiene
Chinese Academy of Preventive Medicine
Beijing, People's Republic of China

Iron deficiency is frequently characterized as the most common nutritional deficiency in both developing and developed countries. Iron deficiency may arise from blood loss or from nutritional causes. Nutritional iron deficiency results from a persisting inadequacy of iron because one's diet is unable to meet normal physiological needs. The population groups most likely to be at risk are preschool children, women of child-bearing age, and in particular, pregnant women. The iron status of these groups often reflects the iron status of the community at large. In the People's Republic of China, iron-deficiency anemia (IDA) is the most common nutritional deficiency. During the past ten years many surveys and studies concerning anemia have been carried out in selected sites in China.

Iron Status of Children in China

The incidence of nutritional iron-deficiency anemia is rather high among Chinese children. In the early 1980s, the Maternal and Child Health Bureau of the Ministry of Public Health conducted a preliminary survey of the prevalence of nutritional anemia among children in selected Chinese provinces and cities. The red blood count (RBC) level (4,000,000 per mm) and hemoglobin level (12g per dl) were chosen as the criteria for measuring normal iron status. The results appear in Table 3-1.[1]

The survey found a high prevalence of anemia. However, this result could have been due to the high standard that was used. In order to assess the prevalence of IDA in certain areas of Beijing, we determined hemoglobin content, RBC, and percentage of hematocrit among children in both urban and rural areas. The 1980–81 survey covered 1,481 children under seven years of age enrolled in sixteen kindergartens and nurseries in urban areas; and 1,757 preschool children in rural areas surrounding the city.[2] The results indicated there was a strong positive correlation among hemoglobin content, RBC, the percentage of hematocrit, and the prevalence of anemia. Table 3-2 contains these results.

Table 3-1

Anemia Prevalence in Preschool Children in Sixteen Provinces and Cities

Area	Total	Urban			Rural		
		Children	Anemics		Children	Anemics	
	(No.)	(No.)	(No.)	(%)	(No.)	(No.)	(%)
South	7,640	3,188	1,777	55.7	2,079	2,052	98.7
Middle	10,779	8,587	5,503	64.1	1,512	1,250	82.7
North	10,811	8,453	3,421	40.5	2,358	1,083	45.9
Total	29,230	20,228	10,701	52.9	5,949	4,385	73.7

Source: Maternal and Child Health Bureau of the Ministry of Public Health and Hematological Group of the Department of Pediatrics in the First Hospital of the Beijing Medical University; Data Collection of the National Children's Nutritional Anemia Training Course, 1981.

The survey revealed that the anemia rates of urban children in a residential kindergarten setting and those who live at home were 8.3 percent and 17.8 percent, respectively. On the other hand, 24.2 percent of the children living in the rural areas surrounding Beijing were found to be anemic. Thus, anemia was more prevalent among the children living in the rural and suburban areas. Among the different age groups, the highest rates were found in children between seven months and two years of age. A dietary survey, using the three-day food weighing method, of children in two nurseries in urban Beijing, showed that the iron intakes of these children averaged only 8.6 mg per day, an amount far below the recommended daily allowance (RDA). In contrast, the iron intakes of children in the kindergarten averaged 12.8 mg per day, an amount that is above the RDA. Therefore, the anemia rate of children in the kindergarten was significantly lower. The results suggested that the cause of IDA in preschool children in Beijing could be due to inadequate iron intakes.

In 1987 Wang et. al. investigated the iron status of 4,747 preschool children in six different areas of China.[3] The diagnosis of IDA is based on hemoglobin (Hb) below the standard and on abnormalities in two out of three measurements of free

Table 3-2

Anemia Prevalence in Preschool Children in Beijing

Age	In Residential Nurseries in Urban Areas			Living at Home in Urban Areas			Living at Home in Suburban Areas		
	Children (No.)	Anemics (No.)	(%)	Children (No.)	Anemics (No.)	(%)	Children (No.)	Anemics (No.)	(%)
>7m	21	2	9.5	211	22	10.4	91	29	31.8
7m–1y	67	24	35.8	207	40	19.3	129	63	48.8
1–2y	234	68	29.1	358	87	24.3	405	149	36.8
2–3y	418	28	6.1	136	14	10.2	252	67	26.6
Subtotal	740	122	16.5	912	163	17.8	877	308	35.1
3–4y	230	1	0.4	–	–	–	201	53	26.4
4–7y	510	8	1.6	–	–	–	679	65	9.6
Total	1,480	131	8.3	–	–	–	1,757	426	24.2

Source: Wang Wen-guang et al., "Studies on Iron-Deficiency Anemia of Preschool Children. 1. A Survey of Iron Deficiency Anemia among Preschool Children in Beijing," *Acta Nutrimenta Sinica* 5, no. 1 (1983): 73–78.

Note: Hemoglobin level below 11 grams per deciliter.

erythrocytes porphyrin (FEP), serum ferritin (SF), and FEP/Hb. The IDA prevalence rates appear in Table 3-3.

Table 3-3

Prevalence of Iron-Deficiency Anemia in Preschool Children in Six Provinces in the People's Republic of China

Age	Beijing	Heilong-jiang	Jiangsu	Xinjiang	Yunnan	Zheiang
6m	32.4	30.0	20.6	29.3	40.8	25.5
1y	18.2	24.6	9.3	32.7	35.0	15.7
2y	18.5	6.2	4.6	20.3	19.3	13.5
3–6y	11.2	4.0	1.0	11.4	12.5	7.7
Average	16.4	10.2	9.4	20.1	24.0	15.3

Source: Wang Wen-guang et al., "Studies of the Relationship between Iron Status and Dietary Patterns in Preschool Children," *Acta Nutrimenta Sinica* 11, no. 3 (1989): 246.

Table 3-3 shows that the anemia prevalence rate in Beijing in 1987 was lower than the results derived in 1981. The analysis of dietary intakes of these children revealed that in the areas where the animal food intake was higher, there was a lower anemia rate. For example, the animal food intake of children in Jiangsu represented 22 percent of the total food intake, the highest proportion among the six areas studied. The protein intake of these children was 79 percent of the RDA. The anemia rate in this area was the lowest, 9.4 percent. In contrast, the anemia rates in Xinjiang and Yunnan were 20.1 percent and 24.0 percent respectively, and animal food intake was only 7 to 8 percent of the total food intake. The data also showed that the children's growth rate was hindered by anemia in each of the six areas. In the areas in which the anemia rate was low, the children's growth rate was higher.

Iron Status of Women in China

The incidence of IDA in pregnant women in China also is quite high: during the first trimester, 1 to 9 percent; in the second trimester, 14 to 24 percent; and in the third trimester, 15 to 26 percent. The incidence of iron deficiency (ID) is even higher than the incidence of IDA: 35 percent and 49 percent in the second and third trimester, respectively. In 1983, Wang et al., conducted an iron nutritional status survey of 645 pregnant women in the Xuan-Wu district of Beijing.[4] Table 3-4 presents the results. The prevalence of anemia tended to increase as pregnancy progressed, with the highest rate occurring in the last trimester, an average rate of 14.9 percent.

Table 3-4

Changes in Hemoglobin, Red Blood Cell, and Hematocrit During Pregnancy

	Trimester		
	First	**Second**	**Third**
Hemoglobin (grams/deciliter)	14.3 ± 1.5	12.5 ± 1.4	12.5 ± 1.6
Red blood cell count ($10,000/mm^3$)	461 ± 47	409 ± 58	409 ± 49
Hematocrit (%)	39 ± 5	35 ± 4	35 ± 4
Iron-deficiency anemia (%)	0.9	13.7	14.9

Source: Wang Wen-quang et al., "Studies on Iron-Deficiency Anemia of Pregnant Women in Beijing," *Acta Nutrimenta Sinica* 6, no. 2 (1984): 135.
Notes: The data shown are the mean values, plus or minus one standard deviation. Hemoglobin concentration is a biochemical parameter used in evaluation of iron nutritional status. Red blood cell count is also a parameter used in evaluation of iron nutritional status. Hematocrit is a relatively insensitive index of mild degrees of iron depletion.

Table 3-5

Changes in Hematologic Parameters of Pregnant Women

	Control	Pregnant Women	
		Second Trimester	**Third Trimester**
	($N = 68$)	($N = 99$)	($N = 89$)
Hemoglobin (grams/deciliter)	13.46 ± 1.28	11.4 ± 1.17	11.3 ± 1.24
Red blood cell count ($10,000/mm^3$)	429 ± 35	369 ± 33	382 ± 39
Free erythrocytes porphyrin (micrograms/deciliter)	38.4 ± 1.4	47.9 ± 1.6	66.8 ± 1.6
Serum ferritin (nanograms/deciliter)	46.2 ± 2.0	10.5 ± 3.8	10.0 ± 3.8

Source: Wang Heng et al., "Study on Iron-Deficiency Anemia during Pregnancy in Beijing," *Acta Nutrimenta Sinica* 10, no. 3 (1988): 201–08.
Notes: The data shown are the mean values, plus or minus one standard deviation. An increase in free erythrocytes porphyrin (FEP) is a sensitive indicator of iron deficiency. The level of serum ferritin (SF) reflects iron stored in the body. This level can be used as a reliable and simple indicator of early iron deficiency.

Table 3-6

Prevalence of Iron-Deficiency Anemia (IDA) and Iron
Deficiency (ID) in Pregnant Women in Beijing

	Second Trimester (N=99)		Third Trimester (N=89)	
	IDA	ID	IDA	ID
Number	34	35	32	44
Rate (%)	34.3	35.4	36.0	49.4

Source: Wang Heng et al., "Study on Iron-Deficiency Anemia during Pregnancy in Beijing,"
Acta Nutrimenta Sinica 10, no. 3 (1988): 201–08.

A similar survey in the city of Harbin showed that the anemia prevalence rates in pregnant women in the second and third trimester were 23.7 percent and 26.0 percent, respectively.[5] A longitudinal study of iron status and dietary iron intake of one hundred pregnant women was carried out in 1985 by one of my colleagues at the Institute of Nutrition and Food Hygiene.[6] The study found a progressive decline in Hb, serum iron (SI), and transferrin saturation (TS) values as pregnancy progressed, and a significant decrease in SF with a rise in FEP. These results appear in tables 3-5 and 3-6.

Nutrient intake of these pregnant women also were inadequate, except for vitamin C, vitamin B1, and iron. Intake of other nutrients also was below the RDA. Table 3-6 shows that the iron status of these pregnant women was poor. In 1987, another study of women living near seven nutritional surveillance sites showed that 24 to 50 percent of the pregnant and the lactating women were suffering from anemia.[7]

Prevention of Iron-Deficiency Anemia

The etiology of IDA is multifaceted. For example, dietary iron content can match the RDA, yet a low hemoglobin level and IDA can still exist. From numerous reports on iron deficiency, a major recent preventive study revealed the main causes of IDA as follows:

1. Lack of knowledge of appropriate dietary content;

2. Insufficient amount of animal protein in the diet and insufficient utilization of heme iron, found principally in animal products;

3. Poor absorption and bioavailability of iron resulting from food intake. Iron in these cases derives predominantly or totally from cereals and from vegeta-

bles (i.e., nonheme iron consisting mainly of iron salts). The absorption of non-heme iron may be decreased by the presence of phytic acid, tannic acid, or oxalic acid, all of which can interfere with the absorption of trace metals, including iron;

4.   Low breast-feeding rate;

5.   Inadequate production of iron-rich supplementary foods and few varieties available on the market;

6.   Poor nourishment during pregnancy, including insufficient iron intake.

China has adopted the following policies regarding breast-feeding, dietary balance, and iron supplementation to combat IDA:

1.   Breast-feeding is to be encouraged, especially in urban areas. Data indicates that the incidence of IDA among breast-fed infants under six months of age was 33 percent, as compared to a rate of 76 percent among bottle-fed children. The statistical difference between the two groups is highly significant (x =25, $p<0.005$).[8]

2.   A well-balanced diet is to be made available to kindergarten children. In 1987, an investigation by Wang, et al., showed that a well-balanced diet can lead to increased physical growth.[9] The study data prior to and after nine weeks of sustained dietary intervention showed significant differences not only in the values for height and body weight of the children, but also for hemoglobin levels. The mean Hb had increased from 10.8 to 11.4 g per dl (t=2.67, $p<0.05$).

3.   Children's diets will include an increased protein content, especially soy bean protein. Studies have revealed that protein intake lower than RDA is an important cause of iron deficiency. Analysis of the diet of IDA children indicated that the agincine and histidine in their diet was lower than that in normal children's diets ($p<0.01$).

4.   Iron supplementation is to be utilized for the treatment of IDA, especially in pregnant women. Where there is a high prevalence of IDA in the population, iron supplementation will be needed to treat the most severely affected individuals. Supplementation is the only way to improve iron status in a relatively short period of time, such as the time period characteristic of pregnancy.

Iron Supplementation

A ferrous iron-fortified sugar supplementation, in a pilot test, was given orally to thirty-three anemic pregnant women. Each received on a daily basis elementary iron of 12.4 mg and ascorbic acid of 66 mg during one month. At the end of the experiment, the mean Hb and HCT values of these subjects were all significantly higher than the values indicated at the beginning of the test. These results are shown in Table 3-7.

In 1986 Wang et al. reported that with a dosage of 2 mg per kg per day given to pregnant women with anemia, the prevalence of anemia could be lowered from 26 percent to 2.5 percent after one month of medication. As for children, the supplementation trial by Wang, et al., also showed good results.[10] The mean Hb, RBC, and HCT values before and after treatment are shown in Table 3-8

Table 3-7

Supplementation in Thirty-Three Anemic Pregnant Women in Beijing

	Before trial	After trial	*p*
Hemoglobin (grams/deciliter)	10.3 ± 0.6	11.7 ± 1.4	< 0.001
Red blood cell count ($10,000/mm^3$)	380 ± 44	394 ± 50	=0.054
Hematocrit (%)	31.6 ± 2.8	33.4 ± 3.6	< 0.002

Source: Wang Wen-guang et al., "Studies on Iron-Deficiency Anemia of Pregnant Women in Beijing," *Acta Nutrimenta Sinica* 6, no. 2 (1984):135–39.

All the children with anemia responded favorably to oral iron and to ascorbic acid administration. The increase in hematology values was statistically significant. Therapeutic daily doses were varied among the children in the study. Some children received 10 mg; others, 20 mg, and yet others, 30 mg daily. Yet the increases in the hematologic values were shown to be similar (see Table 3-8). It is believed, therefore, that 10 mg of elemental iron per day administered by mouth is sufficient to cure IDA in preschool children. The test results of the last two groups also indicate that ascorbic acid supplementation can increase the therapeutic effect of iron in the treatment of IDA. The routine therapeutic dosage of oral iron typically is 5–6 mg per kg per day, but in Wang's experience, a smaller dosage will obtain the same result.[11] In this study of forty-six children with IDA who were given a dosage of 1 mg per kg per day for forty days, hemoglobin levels equivalent to or exceeding the normal values were observed in forty-one cases (89.1 percent) and with a net gain to hemoglobin over 2.0 g per dl in twenty-four cases (52.2 percent).

Since the supplementation approach involves the distribution of hematinic (iron) in tablet form or, in the case of infants and young children, in liquid form, a major problem with the supplementation program is developing and financing an effective distribution mechanism. Distribution channels in different parts of the People's Republic include kindergartens, schools, antenatal clinics, and maternal and child health centers. Since it is difficult to determine consistently whether the dosages are administered in a timely way, it is often difficult to predict results with a high degree of accuracy.

Table 3-8

Therapeutic Effect of Iron Preparations and Ascorbic Acid on Anemic Children

Treatment	Children (N)	Iron intake (mg/day)	Period (month[s])	Before treatment			After treatment		
				Hemoglobin (grams/deciliter)	Red blood cell count (10^4/mm^3)	Hematocrit (%)	Hemoglobin (grams/deciliter)	Red blood cell count (104/mm^3)	Hematocrit (%)
0.3% ferric ammonium citrate	20	10	2	9.6	348	34	12.0	383	39
0.6% ferric ammonium citrate	10	20	2	10.6	372	36	12.0	395	41
1% ferric sulfate	10	30	2	9.7	363	35	12.0	396	42
ascorbic acid	10	0	1	9.7	352	34	11.0	385	37
0.3% ferric ammonium citrate and ascorbic acid	15	10	1	11.0	385	37	12.7	407	42

Source: Wang Wen-guang, Liu Dong-sheng, et al., "Studies on Iron-Deficiency Anemia of Preschool Children. II. Therapeutic Effect of Iron, Ascorbic Acid, and Iron-Fortified Soft Drink Powder in the Treatment of Iron-Deficiency Anemia," *Acta Nutrimenta Sinica* 5, no. 1 (1983):79.

Iron Fortification

Iron fortification of food, increasingly practiced in recent decades, has been found to be an effective means to prevent IDA. The vehicles that are utilized for fortification are the following.

Soft Drink Powder

In 1983, China developed a soft drink powder with a sweet and sour plum taste. This drink is fortified with ferrous sulphate (450 mg) and ascorbic acid (270 mg per 100) for the treatment of IDA among preschool children. A child taking 10 g of the powder on a daily basis received 9 mg of iron and 27 mg of ascorbic acid. The results are shown in table 3-9 and 3-10.

Table 3-9

Therapeutic Effect of Iron-Fortified Soft Drink Powder Given in Beijing Nurseries to Children Under Three Years

Duration (months)	Children (N)	Hemoglobin (grams/deciliter)	Hematocrit (%)
Before treatment			
1	16	10.4	34
2	23	10.6	33
After treatment			
1	16	13.1	38
2	23	14.3	41

Source: Wang Wen-guang, Liu Dong-sheng, et al., "Studies on Iron-Deficiency Anemia of Pre-school Children. II. Therapeutic Effect of Iron, Ascorbic Acid, and Iron-Fortified Soft Drink Powder in the Treatment of Iron-Deficiency Anemia," *Acta Nutrimenta Sinica* 5, no. 1 (1983): 79–84.

Sixteen nursery children with anemia were given the fortified soft drink powder daily for one month. The resulting increase in Hb, RBC, and HCT was significant ($p<0.001$). Another twenty-three children were given the fortified powder for two months, and the increase in Hb and HCT values was even higher than for the children who were given the supplement for only a single month. Children living at home also were given the fortified powder for a three-month period. The mean Hb and HCT values of all the children increased significantly ($p<0.001$). It should be noted that the therapeutic dosage of the elemental iron used in the study (3 mg per kg of body weight) was lower than what is recommended by the World Health

Organization. Currently, this soft drink powder is being produced in food factories and is available in the market.

Table 3-10

Therapeutic Effect of Iron-Fortified Soft Drink Powder Given at Home for Three Months to Children Under Three Years

Groups by hemoglobin level	Children	Iron Intake	Hemoglobin	Hematocrit
(grams/ deciliter)	(N)	(mg/day)	(grams/deciliter)	(%)
Before treatment				
< 11	11	9.1	10.0	32
< 11–12	17	8.6	11.3	34
> 12	73	6.5	12.1	38
After treatment				
< 11	11	9.1	15.1	45
< 11–12	17	8.6	15.0	45
> 12	73	6.5	15.0	44

Source: Wang Wen-guang, Liu Dong-sheng, et al., "Studies on Iron-Deficiency Anemia of Preschool Children. II. Therapeutic Effect of Iron, Ascorbic Acid, and Iron-Fortified Soft Drink Powder in the Treatment of Iron-Deficiency Anemia," *Acta Nutrimenta Sinica* 5, no. 1 (1983): 79–84.

Fortified Weaning Foods and Breads

In the People's Republic all foods produced for infants and children such as infant formulas (i.e., based on cow or other animal milk or else derived from soy bean) and weaning foods (i.e., based on cereals or legumes) are fortified with various forms and dosages of iron, according to national standards for infants and children.

Rusks (e.g., sweet breads) and biscuits are cereal-based, baked foods specifically designed for infants and children. These foods may be used directly or else in pulverized form with the addition of water, milk, or other suitable liquids. Last year a nutritious rusk was produced in two cities of China. Production is under the supervision of the Institute of Nutrition and Food Hygiene, Chinese Academy of Preventive Medicine. The United Biscuits Corporation supplied the recipe. This type of rusk was specially designed for infants by Chinese and British nutrition specialists. It is fortified with three minerals (calcium, iron, and zinc) and seven vitamins. Each piece of rusk provides 5 mg iron; therefore, babies under two years old and children from two to ten can with two and three pieces, respectively, fully satisfy their need for minerals and vitamins, excluding vitamin C. It is an ideal weaning food. This fortification experiment is still in progress, as three food factories in three different provinces shortly will begin producing the rusk.

Chinese Soy Sauce Fortification

Soy sauce is a dark brown liquid that has been used in China for thousands of years. It is consumed daily by every Chinese family. It is added during cooking, especially to pork, fish, chicken, and to some vegetables. It is centrally processed. Thus, it could be an ideal vehicle for iron fortification. In 1983, Dai studied the possibilities of iron fortification of soy sauce.[12] His results, during the course of 16 weeks of observation, showed that iron, in the form of ferrous sulphate, added to Chinese soy sauce in concentrations up to 75 to 100 mg per dl, exhibited good solubility. There were no significant changes in pH or in iron content, and no detectable changes in organoleptic characteristics.

Table 3-11

Absolute Amount of Iron Absorbed from Soy Sauce at a Forty Percent Reference Dose

	Iron Intake	Absorption	Absolute absorption	Iron absorption at 40% reference dose	
	(mg)	(%)	(mg)	(mg)	(%)
Soy sauce	3.0	6.95	0.21	0.32	10.80
Iron-fortified soy sauce	23.0	4.36	1.00	1.56	6.78
Iron-fortified soy sauce and ascorbic acid	23.0	8.35	1.92	2.98	12.98
Reference dose	3.0	25.73	0.77	1.20	40.00

Source: Yua-tian Dai, "Iron Fortification of Chinese Soy Sauce," *Food and Nutrition Bulletin* 5 no. 1 (1983):35–42.

The absorption studies were performed on thirty-one healthy adult volunteers using extrinsic tags of ^{55}Fe and ^{59}Fe. The results revealed that the geometric mean iron absorption from unfortified soy sauce was 6.95 percent and the absolute amount absorbed was 0.21 mg, whereas the iron absorption from iron-fortified soy sauce was 4.36 percent with an absolute amount of absorbed iron of 1.0 mg. Further, it was found that iron absorption from iron-fortified soy sauce, with ascorbic acid added, increased to 8.35 percent, and the absolute amount of iron absorbed amounted to 1.92. (See Table 3-11.) Iron absorption from a vegetable meal containing iron-fortified soy sauce was 5.65 percent, and the absolute amount absorbed was 0.5 mg. Use of pork enhanced the absorption rate by 71 percent, and the absolute amount absorbed increased to 1.08 mg. Green tea inhibited the absorption rate by 84 percent, and diminished the absolute amount of absorbed iron to 0.27 mg. The effects of tea and of meat were highly significant statistically ($p < 0.01$). (See Table 3-12.)

Table 3-12

Absolute Amount of Iron Absorbed from Vegetable Meals Containing Iron-Fortified Soy Sauce at a Reference Dose Absorption of Forty Percent

	Iron content	Absorption	Absolute absorption	Iron absorption at 40% reference dose	
	(mg)	(%)	(mg)	(%)	(mg)
Vegetable meal	8.9	5.65	0.50	6.36	0.57
Vegetable meal and tea	8.9	3.07	0.27	3.46	0.31
Vegetable meal and meat	11.2	9.67	1.08	10.89	1.22
Reference dose	3.0	35.52	1.06	40.00	1.20

Source: Yua-tian Dai, "Iron Fortification of Chinese Soy Sauce," *Food and Nutrition Bulletin* 5 no. 1 (1983):35.

From the above results, it can be argued that the fortification of soy sauce is an effective measure for preventing the development of IDA. Outside the People's Republic, soy sauce also is widely used in Japan, Korea, and some countries of Southeast Asia. Therefore, iron-fortified soy sauce could be used in these countries as well. In all, approximately one-third of the world's population could benefit from the use of iron-fortified soy sauce in preventing iron deficiency.

Fortified Salt

Using table salt as a vehicle for iron fortification is a proven way to prevent IDA. In 1988 Ho observed the effect of using iron-fortified salt at the level of 5 to 10 mg of iron supplement.[13] The test involved preschool children in Xinghui county of Guang Dong Province. Two groups of children residing in different kindergartens were the subjects. One group was given the fortified salt and the other served as control group during a period of one year. The initial hemoglobin levels of both groups were the same. However, one year later, the hemoglobin level of the experimental group had changed from 11.78 0.57 g per dl up to 12.72 0.70 g per dl, and became significantly different from that of the control group ($p<0.05$). The iron-fortified salt consumption did not cause any side effects in the children. It was found to be an effective means for preventing anemia in a suitable setting.

In Sichuang province, Liao added ferrous sulphate to table salt in concentrations of 1 mg of elementary iron per gram.[14] Kindergarten children with IDA were treated with iron-fortified salt for a period of three months. The hemoglobin levels of these children increased significantly ($p<0.001$): from an average of 11.03 g per dl prior to treatment to 13.2 g per dl after treatment. Salt is consumed universally by most population groups in China and iron-fortified table salt was found to be of particular benefit in rural, underdeveloped, and inaccessible areas. Fortified salt was shown to be of advantage in treating and preventing IDA, because it is a safe, economical, and practical approach, even in remote areas.

Conclusion

China's experience in combatting IDA and other nutritional disorders points to the central role of nutrition education. Nutrition training and education provide pregnant women and mothers with the information necessary to protect the health of their children. It is a key to understanding the need for healthful diets, especially for the very young and, wherever necessary, the appropriate uses of food supplementation and fortification techniques in both the prevention and treatment of nutritional disorders. Education also is a key to training and developing health care and nutrition professionals, as well as volunteer workers, who constitute the front line in safeguarding household and community health.

In conclusion, the experience and expertise of physicians, pediatricians, health care professionals, and nutritionists in China leads to the following recommendations in treating iron deficiency in children and in women: 1) make every effort to encourage breast-feeding; 2) whenever necessary, commence iron supplementation in infancy, and continue this course for one to three years duration; 3) use appropriate types of food supplements, including iron-rich foods and iron-fortified foods, as well as supplemental tablets and liquid dosages; 4) and increase the consumption of ascorbic-acid, vitamin C-rich foods such as fresh fruits, or the equivalent in tablet or liquid form.

Once IDA is diagnosed, the etiology has to be examined and identified, so that an appropriate course of treatment can be undertaken. This course of treatment, generally, should be of sufficient duration, at a minimum of a period of one to three months, so as to provide for a buildup of iron while the Hb level returns to a normal status.

Notes

1. Unpublished data from a joint study conducted for the National Children's Nutritional Anemia Training Course by the Maternal and Child Health Bureau of the Ministry of Public Health and the Hematological Group of the Department of Pediatrics in the First Hospital of the Beijing Medical University, 1981.

2. Wang Wen-guang et al., "Studies on Iron-deficiency Anemia of Preschool Children I: A Survey of Iron-deficiency Anemia among Preschool Children in Beijing," *Acta Nutrimenta Sinica* 5:1 (1983):73–78.

3. Wang Wen-guang et al., "Studies of the Relationship between Iron Status and Dietary Patterns in Preschool Children," *Acta Nutrimenta Sinica* 11:3 (1989):246–49.

4. Wang Wen-guang et al., "Studies on Iron-deficiency Anemia of Pregnant Women in Beijing," *Acta Nutrimenta Sinica* 6:2 (1984):135–39.

5. Hou Penjie et al., "A Nutrition Survey of Pregnant Women in Harbin City," *Acta Nutrimenta Sinica* 6:2 (1984):141ff.

6. Wang Heng et al., "Study on Iron-deficiency Anemia During Pregnancy in Beijing," *Acta Nutrimenta Sinica* 10:3 (1988):201–08.

7. Liu Dong-sheng, "Nutrition Surveillance Project of the Institute of Nutrition and Food Hygiene," Chinese Academy of Preventive Medicine, 1987 (unpublished).

8. Zhou Z. Z. et al., "Measurements of Iron Status," *Child Food Science Society Guidelines* (Beijing, 1988), pp. 191, 193, 207, 208.

9. Wang R. W. et al., "An Investigation on Iron Status Among 854 Children," *Journal of Chinese Hematology* 12 (1987).

10. Wang Wen-guang et al., "Studies on Iron-deficiency Anemia of Preschool Children II: Therapeutic Effect of Iron, Ascorbic Acid and Iron Fortified Soft Drink Powder in the Treatment of Iron-deficiency Anemia," *Acta Nutrimenta Sinica* 5:1 (1983):79–84; Wang Wen-guang, Chen Xue-cun, and Liu Dong-sheng, "Hematologic Response to Iron and Ascorbic Acid Administration in Preschool Children with Anemia," *Nutrition Research* 6 (1986):241–48.

11. Wang R. W. et al., "A Synchronous Study on the Iron Status of Mothers and Babies," *Journal of Applied Clinical Pediatrics* 1:2 (1986):1–7.

12. Yau-tian Dai, "Iron Fortification of Chinese Soy Sauce," *Food and Nutrition Bulletin*, 5:1 (1983): 35–42.

13. Zhichien Ho et al., "Preliminary Study of Preventing Iron-deficiency Anemia by Iron Fortification of Table Salt," *ACTA Nutrimenta Sinica*, 10:1 (1988): 46–49.

14. Liao Qing-Kui et al., "The Treatment and Prevention of Children's Iron-deficiency Anemia," *Chinese Journal of Hematology*, 7:7 (1986): 389.

CHAPTER 4

Food and Nutrition Security in East, Central, and Southern Africa: A Study of Two Regional Initiatives

Tshire O. Maribe
Chief Nutritionist, Ministry of Health
Gaborone, Republic of Botswana

African food and nutrition problems have received extensive consideration. Substantial efforts to alleviate suffering and to improve the quality of life have been made. Yet childhood malnutrition and hunger continue to increase. The question is, why? The response to this question has much to do with the continuing, unresolved problems affecting African food systems. It is essential in assessing the possibilities of improving the food and nutrition situation in Africa to consider the existing human and institutional capacities, if positive changes are to be realized.

In this connection, two organizations bear examination. Both operate in the southern, eastern, and central regions of Africa, and their work is of major consequence in improving the conditions of food and nutrition in Africa. These organizations are building the capacity to meet the basic requirements of effective food and nutrition programs. They will play a key role in raising public and official awareness of the relationship between nutrition and food security, on the one hand, and solving the problems of hunger and malnutrition, on the other. Sadly, as the August 1990 report of the Southern Africa Development Coordination Conference (SADCC) acknowledges, there is currently a dearth of understanding of the concept of food security and too little recognition of its importance even in the education and training of professionals who plan to work in the fields of health, nutrition, and food policy.[1]

The case study of two multinational, regional organizations in Africa and their cooperative initiatives in combatting hunger and malnutrition can provide other nations and regions of Africa with useful models for the design and implementation of yet other food and nutrition security programs.

Figure 4-1

Organizational Model for Regional Food and Nutrition Programming

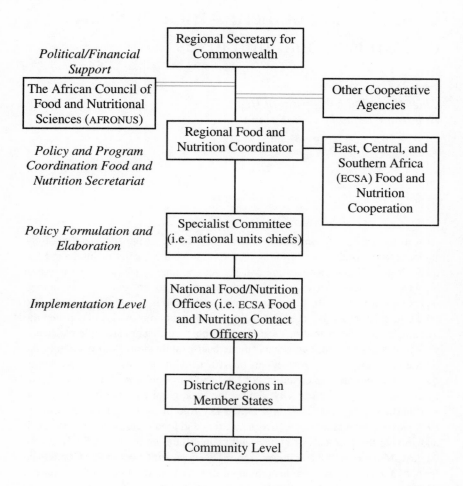

Source: African Council of Food and Nutritional Sciences (AFRONUS), Dar-es-Salaam, Tanzania, 1988.

Food and Nutrition Initiatives

The two institutions are the East, Central, and Southern Africa Food and Nutrition Cooperation (ECSA) and the Southern Africa Development Coordination Conference (SADCC). Table 4-1 identifies the members of these two organizations. The first is made up of eleven Commonwealth and four non-Commonwealth countries; while the latter is made up of ten of these fifteen countries.

Figure 4-1 shows the structure for organizing regional food and nutrition planning. The double lines signify the plans to develop future collaborative relationships with other regional bodies. The strong similarities should be noted between the food and nutrition programs of ECSA and some of the program components of the Food Security Sector of SADCC.[2] Not all ECSA countries fall within the SADCC region but this does not diminish the potential to develop complementary project linkages that can be of great benefit in improving country and regional food systems.

Food and Nutrition Situation

The January-March 1990 *Food Security Bulletin* of SADCC indicates that, at the regional level, domestic food availability is expected to be 106 percent of the total requirements.[3] Despite this impressive position, the majority of these countries continue to experience food insecurity at both the national and household levels (see Table 4-2). Even in those countries with net surpluses, problems of access to food are being experienced at the household level among significant population groups. Malnutrition ranges from 11 percent in Zimbabwe to a range of 27 to 56 percent in Malawi, indicating the magnitude of the problem of food accessibility. The incidence of malnutrition highlights the need for ECSA cooperation to address food security as the challenge of the 1990s and beyond.

An Operational Framework

Structures, mechanisms, and procedures exist at the national level that are designed to address the multisectoral nature of nutrition problems. However, the sophistication of these structures varies by country. In a number of the countries the lack of monitoring and evaluation has diminished the improvements that otherwise could be made.

Studies indicate that Malawi, Kenya, and Botswana are the only countries in the region that have policy coordinating units within the central planning agencies with the specific mandate to bring together the different policy sectors (Table 4-3).[4] In comparative terms this arrangement seems to work more effectively than other mechanisms since the responsibility of these units is strictly coordinative, in contrast to mechanisms that combine implementation and coordination. The latter tend to get more involved in operational issues due largely to the placement of responsibility in a line ministry.

Table 4-1

Countries by Cooperative Organization

Country	Organization	
	East, Central, and Southern Africa (ECSA) Food and Nutrition Cooperation	**Southern Africa Development Coordination Conference (SADCC)**
Angola	X	X
Botswana	X	X
Ethiopia	X	–
Kenya	X	–
Lesotho	X	X
Malawi	–	X
Mauritius	X	–
Mozambique	X	X
Namibia	X	X
Seychelles	X	–
Somalia	X	–
Sudan	X	–
Tanzania	X	X
Uganda	X	–
Zambia	X	X
Zimbabwe	X	X

N. M. Lenneiye identifies seven such institutional arrangements (Table 4-3) and analyzes the strength and the weakness of these structures.[5] For example, communication was found to be the single most important factor that explains the effectiveness of these mechanisms. Improvements resulting from specific program interventions have been shown in some of these countries, as health indicators demonstrate. However, further improvements in conditions can only come about by actions taken in the other sectors besides health and through activities targeted to the underserved and to remote rural areas. This suggests that ministries of agriculture, among others, also have to assume a leading role in program development if further improvements are to be made.

The following operational framework should form the basis for guiding the planning and implementation of food and nutrition programs:

1. Continued improvements in nutritional status must become explicit objectives of development policies and of planning at the national, district, and village levels;

2. District-specific frameworks and the design of locality-specific interventions are crucial and should reflect the decentralized government structure in many of these countries;

3. Food and nutrition surveillance activities for planning, monitoring, advocacy, and early warning purposes should be established in all the countries, and existing systems strengthened;

4. Food and nutrition information should be developed for use at the village level. Such development is vitally important in providing an entry point for community involvement in food and nutrition programs;

5. The managerial, technical, and analytical competence of staff responsible for implementing programs and projects must be increased;

6. Intersectoral mechanisms for planning, implementing, monitoring, and evaluating programs must be improved and created where they do not presently exist;

7. Macroeconomic policies and development plans should take into account the potential effects on nutrition and health, in particular the effects on the most vulnerable population groups; and remedial actions should be taken, wherever necessary, to improve the food and nutrition situation.

Core Strategies

In 1984 a Regional Specialist Committee determined priority areas that should form the program of cooperation for ECSA.[6] It is ECSA's goal to provide effective regional leadership in country-level programming and to utilize in an adaptive manner the operational framework identified above. Strategies and programs in human resource development, food and nutrition security, nutrition intervention, primary health care, and related areas are being employed in the region, on a priority basis, to deliver food and nutrition services.

Human Resource Development

This area is recognized as a prerequisite for effective and sustainable program development and, thus, given the highest priority. Organizationally, a regionwide subcommittee on training exists, whose ability to organize and manage training programs has been tested and found to be a model for replication by the countries in the region.[7] The Third Africa Food and Nutrition Congress, held in September 1988, passed a resolution urging all governments and donors to give highest

Table 4-2

Balances for Major Staples for 1990–91 Market Year, in Maize-equivalent 1,000 tons

Country	Opening Stock	Production	Total Available[1]	Consumption Requirement	Carryover Requirement	Total Require-ment[2]	Surplus/Deficit[3]	Exports Planned	Imports Planned
Angola	32.7	740.3	773.0	1,234.1	54.1	1,288.2	-515.2	0.0	279.2
Botswana	140.6	52.7	193.3	198.2	0.0	198.2	-4.9	N/A	N/A
Lesotho	55.9	184.4	240.3	362.3	16.4	378.7	-138.4	N/A	N/A
Malawi	233.0	1,453.2	1,686.2	1,647.8	51.6	1,699.4	-13.2	4.0	N/A
Mozambique	31.1	1,710.2	1,741.3	2,126.6	111.4	2,238.0	-496.7	N/A	N/A
Mozambiquean refugees in Malawi	N/A	N/A	N/A	115.0	N/A	115.0	N/A	N/A	N/A
Swaziland	0.0	130.3	130.3	179.0	2.0	181.0	-50.7	N/A	N/A
Tanzania	212.1	7,232.8	7,444.9	5,905.0	306.3	6,211.3	1,233.6	N/A	N/A
Zambia	839.0	1,518.5	2,356.5	1,661.5	225.0	1,886.5	470.0	N/A	N/A
Zimbabwe	1,406.2	2,522.6	3,928.8	2,217.8	687.8	2,906.6	1,022.2	322.8	51.7
SADCC[4] Total	2,950.6	15,545.0	18,495.6	15,697.4	1,454.5	17,151.9	1,343.7	359.8	330.9

Source: SADCC Annual Report, 1989–90. Harare, Zimbabwe.

Notes: "N/A" indicates that data is not available. [1]"Opening Stock" plus "Production" equals "Total Available." [2] "Consumption Requirement" plus "Carryover Requirement" equals "Total Requirement." [3]"Total Available" minus "Total Requirement" equals "Surplus/Deficit." [4] Southern Africa Development Coordination Conference.

priority to technical training and institution building for dealing with food and nutritional problems. The commitment of governments is needed to ensure the appropriate employment of food and nutrition professionals. Throughout the region, governments and private voluntary organizations are finding it increasingly difficult to retain skilled staff.

Table 4-3

Mechanism for Coordinating Food and Nutrition Work by Country

Country	Mechanism					
	Government Commission	Agriculture Ministry	Education Ministry	Health Ministry	Finance and Development Ministry	President or Prime Minister
Botswana				X	X	
Kenya		X	X	X	X	
Lesotho				X		
Malawi		X				X
Namibia				X		
Seychelles			X	X		
Swaziland		X	X			
Tanzania	X	X	X	X		
Zambia	X					
Zimbabwe				X		

Source: N. M. Lenneiye, *Report on Training Needs Assessment for Food and Nutrition Programs in East, Central, and Soluthern Africa Region*, Vol. 1. Gaborone, Botswana: ECSAFAN Cooperation, 1991.

This is an important issue to be addressed in order for human resource development to take effect in building strong African institutions. Regionwide surveys of need assessment, however, have not addressed the training role and its consequences and none of the reports on training have looked at this issue in an adequate way. This does require follow-up, particularly at the country level since training capabilities provide a pivotal point for constructive intervention. A training needs assessment in food and nutrition has been carried out within the region, and Table 4-4 summarizes preliminary data on country-level training initiatives. Some of these training needs have been identified by the Food Studies Group of the Regional Food Reserve Project under SADCC, thus emphasizing the need for stronger collaboration among the cooperating agencies. Meetings held in Lesotho at the end of October 1990 have facilitated the efforts to develop a master plan for regional training.

Household Level Food and Nutrition Security

The regional commitment to improve household-level food security and nutrition is expressed at the highest level, among the heads of state of the SADCC countries. This level of commitment exists alongside the political and financial support that ECSA receives from the health ministers of Commonwealth countries. The planning requirements of both organizations indicate a strong involvement of country-level institutions in developing programs and plans of action. These factors can facilitate the continuous assessment and evaluation of food systems within the respective countries as well the collective determination to pursue remedial strategies. The linkage between National Early Warning Systems and the Regional Early Warning Systems provides an additional avenue for generating much needed information about food and nutrition problems. It is through such means of communication that food production, distribution gaps, and food access problems can be effectively identified. These means have been instrumental in raising awareness of the plight of the most vulnerable population groups and in further operationalizing the concept of "food security." K. J. M. Dhliwayo reiterates this in a SADCC publication: "Through collective analysis of the problems of food insecurity, SADCC member states have continued to sharpen and clearly define their concept of food security."[8] These new policy directions affecting household-level problems are of crucial importance in achieving sustainable improvements in food and nutrition accessibility.

Nutrition Interventions

Program planning and implementation in the area of nutrition interventions continue to be undertaken in the face of human and institutional limitations. One example of a compromised program outcome is the ineffective delivery of services and, as a result, beneficiaries' and policy makers' loss of confidence in program credibility. Yet, there are some successful programs that strongly indicate the need to organize at the country and regional levels. Two examples are especially noteworthy.

Micronutrient Deficiencies
Energy deficiency is an important problem afflicting both the young and the old alike. There are also problems with micronutrient deprivation, whose severity

Table 4-4

Training Initiatives in Selected Member Nations of the East, Central, and Southern Africa (ECSA) Food and Nutrition Cooperation

Country	Formal Training		In-Service Training
	Certificate/Degree	**Institution**	
Botswana	Program Management	Institute of Development Management	Food/Nutrition Surveillance and Early Warning
	Proposed B. Sc., Home Economics	University of Botswana	
Kenya	M. Sc., Applied Nutrition	Kabete Campus	
	Medical Nutrition	Kenyatta University College	
	Home Economics	Egerton College	
Malawi	–	–	Food and Nutrition Policy and Food Aid Management
Swaziland	Food Policy Management	Namanga Training Center	
	Home Economics	University of Swaziland	
Tanzania	B. Sc., Food Science and Technology	Sokoine University of Agriculture	Organization and Management Systems Program Planning in Nutrition
Zambia	–	–	Socioeconomic Analysis
Zimbabwe	Food Service Management	–	Community Nutrition Projects
	Proposed B. Sc., Nutrition	University of Zimbabwe	Institutional Food Service

Source: N. M. Lenneiye, *Report on Training Needs Assessment for Food and Nutrition Programs in East, Central, and Southern Africa Region*, Vol. 1. Gaborone, Botswana: ECSAFAN Cooperation, 1991.

varies by country and within countries. The emerging approach is to undertake a situational analysis in order to generate information for control programs.

The control of iodine-deficiency disorders (IDD) on a regionwide basis is coordinated by Tanzania. IDD studies indicate the prevalence of mild to moderate deficiencies, as well as the existence of problems in specific areas of the affected countries. Salt iodation programs are starting up in Botswana, Kenya, Tanzania, and Namibia. A resolution was passed in Dar-es-Salaam in March 1990 requesting the Government of Botswana to iodate some of the 650,000 tons of salt that are expected to be produced by the Sua Pan Project that is scheduled to start up in June 1991. Discussions are presently underway with the World Health Organization to investigate how this project can meet in-country and regional requirements and thus benefit regional IDD eradication initiatives.

Vitamin A deficiency and iron-deficiency anemia (IDA) are the other disorders whose control is measurable only at national levels. It is recognized, however, that combatting micronutrient deficiencies must be supplemented by an increasing dietary intake of required nutrients. The Malawi project on vitamin A exemplifies this comprehensive approach and is being studied for potential regionwide applications.

Supplementary Feeding

The alleviation of poverty will be a major challenge in the future, affecting the strategies and programs that aim to eliminate hunger and malnutrition. Food supplements will have to be provided on a long-term basis to vulnerable groups. This realization however, is coupled with the recognition that certain aspects of current supplementary food programs will have to be changed. The development and production of weaning foods, currently underway in Botswana, is an example of a shift in policy with respect to the use of donated foods for vulnerable groups. Elsewhere, there are moves to revive traditional techniques for cereal germination and fermentation in the efforts to improve the consumption of local foods by young children.

This approach has numerous economic and social benefits and, above all, has the potential of involving entire communities in the fight against hunger and malnutrition. Community involvement can become more effective than presently, as the Tanzania and Zimbabwean experiences indicate. In Zimbabwe local farmers supply food for a supplementary food production program. These initiatives combine short-, medium-, and long-term objectives into nutrition intervention strategies, thereby building in an element of sustainability.

Food and Nutrition Surveillance

Increasingly, information resources that are linked to decision-making processes are receiving considerable recognition. Within the region ten countries have created some form of food and nutrition surveillance capacity, but only Botswana and Tanzania have established fully operational systems with a wide range of coverage. An FAO paper, presented at the Sixteenth Regional Conference for Africa, noted that the inclusion of a nutrition component in early warning systems, particularly for drought-prone countries, has proven to be very effective in helping to identify the extent and location of food-deficit areas.[9] The Botswana system since its inception in 1984 has had a nutrition component in its early warning system.

President Q. K. J. Masire of Botswana was a recipient of the 1989 Africa Hunger Prize, largely because of his support in developing responsive country-specific information systems that integrate data analysis and decision making, and that link short-term emergency food assistance to long-term development needs. The lessons of this experience have been disseminated in the region and throughout Africa.

Famine Prevention and Management

Even though this is not yet an area of collaboration for ECSA, the countries of the region suffer periodic food-related disasters, including severe drought. Unfortunately, effective response mechanisms still do not exist in many of the affected countries. Botswana, although possessing an excellent capability to deal with droughts, as reflected in the drought experience of 1982–87, still has to evolve a mechanism that integrates drought management with long-term development planning, and that will ensure the "drought proofing" of the rural economy.

Nutrition in Primary Health Care

Table 4-3 indicates that food and nutrition activities are largely the responsibility of the ministries of health where these activities typically come under primary health care or maternal and child health departments. It is, therefore, critical to make a distinction between activities that easily lend themselves to a framework of primary health care, and others that fall outside the health sector itself. Once this categorizing is done, strong program linkages then can be developed to enable a complementary delivery of services, thus promoting program synergy. This is imperative in order to facilitate the creation of strong intersectoral planning mechanisms with clearly defined agendas.

Future Directions

ECSA is only six years old and its structure and program of cooperation still are in their infancy. There is no doubt, however, that its establishment represents a significant achievement, one that clearly expresses a regional need to put into place a framework for cooperative action to guide future planning. This regional framework will continue to expand by expanding ECSA cooperation, encouraging inter-agency collaboration, developing a training master plan, and strengthening national capability.

Strengthening of ECSA Cooperation

Further consolidation of this organization will be done through the establishment of a coordinating office within the Commonwealth Regional Health Secretariat in Arusha, Tanzania. This is a basic requirement that should precede everything else, and it will be accelerated by the recruitment of a regional coordinator.

Interagency Collaboration

Even though emphasis has been given to collaboration between ECSA and SADCC, such activity does not preclude the entry of other organizations that have similar interests. It is critical that strong linkages be developed now. These should capitalize on the momentum that resulted from the tenth anniversary celebration of SADCC's existence held in Gaborone, Botswana, in August 1990. One area for further and more intensified collaboration is training, since it is of major concern to both agencies.

Development of a Training Master Plan

The midterm evaluation of ECSA's regional training experience indicated that with adequate support resources, regional training capabilities are quite possible. The momentum generated in this project's implementation needs to be maintained since it represents an investment in both human and institutional capacity building. Once a master plan for training is developed, project proposals can be prepared for submission to potential donors.

Strengthening of National Capability

Strong country-level institutions have to be developed, as a priority. A major task facing the new regional Food and Nutrition Coordinator is to follow up on country-level institutional development. It is only through optimally functioning and carefully directed national offices that ECSA can be sustained as a strong and effective cooperative structure.

Conclusion

Despite certain capability constraints, there is evidence that successful programs are being planned and implemented under very difficult working conditions. There is evidence, too, that country and regional institutions can first take root in local communities and later at district and national levels and then be linked to regional collaborative efforts. Political commitment exists and all these factors can be pooled together to create a framework for effective action in eliminating hunger and malnutrition. This will, however, remain a desire and a lofty promise unless basic requirements regarding human and institutional needs are met. Therefore, initiatives such as ECSA deserve major support. They represent opportunities for developing effective food and nutrition programs that reflect the pooling of resources and cooperative action among government agencies and among the countries of the region.

Notes

1. *Food Security Programme: Report on Regional Food Reserve Project Training Pre-implementation Study* (Gaborone, Botswana: Southern Africa Development Coordination Conference, 1990).

2. *Report on a Workshop on Household Food Security and Nutrition* (Windhoek, Namibia: United Nations Children's Fund, 1989).

3. *Food Security Bulletin* January–March 1990 (Harare, Zimbabwe: Southern Africa Development Coordination Conference, 1990).

4. *Regional Food Reserve Project: Training Pre-implementation Study* (Gaborone, Botswana: Southern Africa Development Coordination Conference, 1990).

5. N. M. Lenneiye, *Training Needs Assessment for Food and Nutrition Programmes in East, Central, and Southern Africa Region,* Vol. 1 (Gaborone, Botswana, 1991).

6. *Report of the Second Meeting of Regional Nutrition Specialists on Food and Nutrition, Malawi* (Gaborone, Botswana: Commonwealth Regional Health Community for East, Central and Southern Africa, 1985).

7. G. W. Peter, G. Almroth, and J. Kaunda, *Midterm Evaluation of the ECSA Food and Nutrition Courses: Harare, Zimbabwe* (The Hague: Centre for the Study of Education in Developing Countries, 1989).

8. K. J. M. Dhliwayo, *National Food Security Policies and Challenges: SADCC Countries' Experiences* (Harare: University of Zimbabwe, Department of Agricultural Economics, 1989).

9. *Strategies for Combatting Malnutrition in Africa* (Rome: FAO, Food and Agriculture Organization, 1990).

CHAPTER 5

Integrating National Food, Nutrition, and Health Policy: The Chilean Experience

Fernando Monckeberg B.
Director, Institute of Nutrition and Food Technology
University of Chile
Santiago, Chile

During the last thirty years, a progressive and continuous improvement in the health and nutrition of infants and preschool children has taken place in Chile. Biomedical indicators show that Chile has reached one of the highest levels in the region although during this period per capita gross national product (GNP) has not changed substantially. Also during this same period, economic policies have changed drastically, ranging from a planned, centralized economy until 1974, to an open, liberal economy from 1976 until the present. In the last thirty years the county has confronted many severe economic and political crises. A socialist government was overthrown by a military coup in 1973. Two severe economic crises occurred in 1975 and 1982, associated with high unemployment rates which in the latter period reached 20 percent of the total labor force. Despite these numerous changes and crises, malnutrition and infant and preschool child mortality have continued to decrease.[1]

The situation was quite different prior to the early 1960s. Chile had one of the highest infant mortality rates in Latin America (120 per thousand). This decreased to 17 per thousand in 1989, one of the lowest rates in the region (Figure 5-1). This decline in the infant death rate resulted from a remarkable decrease in infant mortality from respiratory and diarrheal disease in children less than one year old (Figure 5-2). A similar trend has been observed in preschool child mortality, that has declined from 14 per thousand in 1960 to 0.8 per thousand in 1989.[2]

At the same time, the percentage of children with malnutrition has also been reduced dramatically, from 37 percent in 1960, to 8.5 percent in 1989. Second- and third-degree malnutrition similarly decreased from 5.9 percent to 0.6 percent (Table 5-1).

Table 5-1

Percentage of Malnourished Children (0–6 Years) in Chile, 1960–1989

Year	Total	Mildly	Moderately	Severely
1960	37.0	31.1	4.1	1.8
1970	19.3	15.8	2.5	1.0
1980	11.5	10.0	1.4	0.2
1989	8.5	7.9	0.5	0.1

Source: Informe Anual, 1990 (Santiago: Ministry of Health), p. 19.

Maternal nutrition has improved if we consider that the percentage of newborns with low birth weight (below 2.5 kg) has diminished from 11.6 percent to 6.4 percent from 1975 to 1988.

Malnutrition, Poverty, and Underdevelopment

It is self-evident that malnutrition is the result of poverty and underdevelopment. Many authors have demonstrated that in any given country there is a close relationship between the level of underdevelopment and the percentage of children suffering from malnutrition. In Chile, however this correlation really does not exist. The nutritional condition of children up to five years of age is much better than the socioeconomic realities of the county would predict (Figure 5-3).

Similarly, studies have shown a close relationship between life expectancy and per capita GNP. Again, this relationship is not observed in the case of Chile, where the life expectancy is much higher than what would be expected from per capita GNP (Figure 5-4).[3]

This anomaly calls for close analysis because it demonstrates that under certain conditions it is possible to improve health and nutrition even when there is no substantial economic development. These facts, as observed in Chile, contradict the claims of many economists who believe that progress in health and nutrition only can be achieved through a substantial degree of sustained economic development. In this view, economic growth creates new resources that permeate the different strata of the society and ultimately improve living conditions, even among the lowest socioeconomic groups.

From our point of view, however, this economic analysis is not plausible because development itself cannot be achieved if a high percentage of the population is already damaged as a consequence of poverty and malnutrition and barely able to survive because of poor health conditions. Malnutrition, poverty, and underdevelopment constitute a truly vicious cycle, which works to hinder economic growth.

Considering these two different points of view and given an environment of limited resources, two different strategies arise for preventing malnutrition and improving health conditions: 1) to focus the effort on achieving large-scale economic growth and development; and 2) to focus efforts on targeted health, nutrition, and education interventions to improve the well-being of the population, especially the most deprived groups.

With respect to the first strategy, one might conclude that if a society were to devote all efforts to economic development and to generating expanded economic resources, then increased wealth would progressively benefit greater numbers of individuals, eventually reaching the entire population. However, two questions

Figure 5-1

Decline in Infant Mortality in Chile from 1940 to 1988

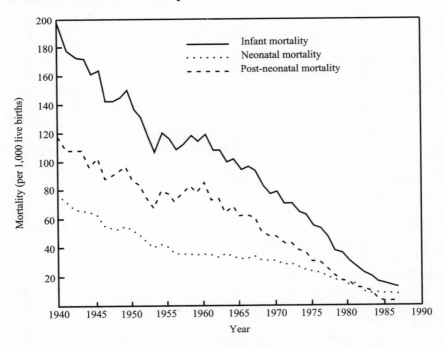

Source: F. Monckeberg, "The Possibilities for Nutrition Intervention," *Food Technology* 35, no. 9 (1981):115.

Note: An infant is a child under one year old. A neonate is a child under one month old. A post-neonate is a child from one month to twelve months old.

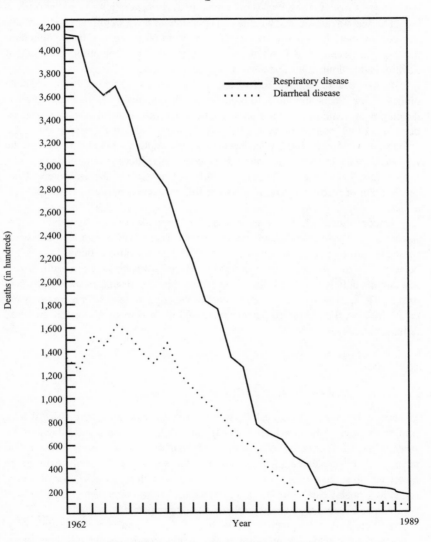

Figure 5-2

Chile: Infant Mortality as a Result of Respiratory and/or Diarrheal Disease, 1962–1989 (per 100,000 live births)

Source: Informe Anual, 1990 (Santiago, Chile: Ministry of Health), p. 12.

Note: The figures for infant mortality reflect the deaths of children twelve months and less.

arise from this approach. The first is, how long would it take under the best circumstances for this wholesale improvement to occur, taking into account the realities existing in poor countries? Poor countries for the most part lack adequate technologies and the wherewithal either for generating or acquiring these technologies. These countries tend to have inefficient infrastructures, lack trained workers, have a low savings capacity, have little investment capital, and to be burdened by a large foreign debt. The logical answer then is that, on the average, economic development would take a long time, probably many generations, to accomplish.

The second question is, whether it is possible to have significant and continuous development in countries in which from 30 to 60 percent of their population has been physically and psychologically damaged over generations as result of poverty and malnutrition. The answer, again, is negative.

If we seek to achieve socioeconomic development, which is the ultimate objective, the essential point is to break out of the vicious cycle created by underdevelopment, malnutrition, and poor health conditions. Human resources are, indeed, one of the most important, albeit insufficiently recognized, factors for social development. Modern society has become very complex, and the demands on the knowledge and skills of its members grow constantly. Incorporating individuals as useful members of the community is really not possible if the environment deprives them of well-being and hinders the full expression of their genetic potentialities.

Under these conditions, even if some economic improvement occurs, it is not likely to reach the lowest socioeconomic strata, where malnutrition and disease is most prevalent. This assertion is confirmed by many observations. During the decade of 1970–80, for example, economic progress was observed in Latin America, but this only led to a widening gap in economic circumstances among different groups. Thus, while the poorest 20 percent of the population did not increase its per capita income, the richest 10 percent increased its income by about four hundred dollars, on an average.[4]

Need for a Political Decision

Protecting the human resources of a country is a difficult, long-term task. At least four areas have to be considered: health, nutrition, sanitation, and education. A strategy has to be adopted to develop the human resources in each of these four areas, and to coordinate programs among the sectors. Individuals have to be protected from the moment they are born or even before, by adequate nutrition, sanitation, health care, education, and housing. These components must be well coordinated because they are interrelated and interdependent.

It is obvious that all nations would benefit from a nutrition and health policy. Yet a universal helth and nutrition policy would require considerable resources, and the ultimate decision rests at the political level. In a situation of underdevelopment, governments have many urgent priorities to confront, and oftentimes political decisions on health and nutrition take a back seat and are postponed. Unfortunately, those who suffer from extreme poverty and malnutrition are not well organized and lack the means to exert political pressure. Furthermore, results take a long time to become visible, and policy makers frequently need to have immediate results.

Figure 5-3

Correlation between Nutritional Status of Children below Six Years of Age and Degree of Development in Selected Countries

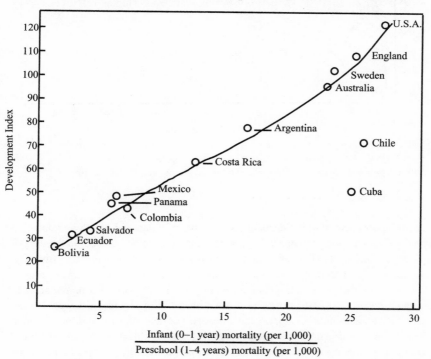

Source: F. Monckeberg, "The Possibilities for Nutrition Intervention," *Food Technology* 35, no. 9 (1981):115.

Note: Degree of development has been calculated using an indicator developed by the Institute of Social Development of the United Nations, based on eighty different items. Lower numbers indicate less development. The infant and preschool mortality rates have been selected as indicators of nutritional status.

Figure 5-4

Life Expectancy in Relation to GNP

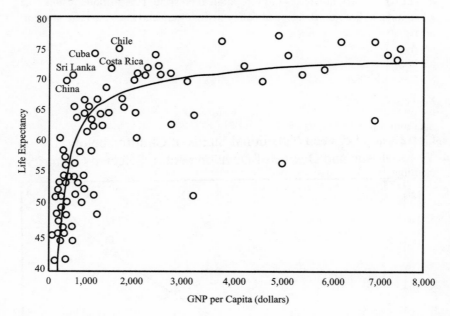

GNP per Capita (dollars)

Source: UNICEF Commission on Health Research Development, *Health Research: Essential Link to Equity in Development* (New York: Oxford University Press, 1990), p. 10.

Note: Line of central tendency is a freehand curve.

In my experience, political decisions supportive of a national health and nutrition policy do not happen spontaneously; rather, they have to be induced. In the case of Chile, the university (Universidad de Chile) and especially our institute (Instituto de Nutrición y Tecnologia des los Alimentos, or INTA) have played a very important role. Talking very pragmatically, while the first priority of a politician is to achieve power, the first priority of a government is to remain in power. On the basis of this assumption, support for a desired political decision will be obtained only when the decision will bring benefits to the political supporters. In other words, to provoke a favorable political decision, malnutrition and health problems have to become visible political issues.

For many years we have developed a defined communications strategy to create awareness of nutritional and health problems in the community. With this purpose in mind, we have utilized for years the mass media, even the training of journalists, in an attempt to create awareness about the adverse effects of malnutrition and poor health upon individuals and the whole society.

Only when this communications stage has been reached will politicians become disposed to incorporate health and nutrition programs or interventions into their political platforms. Although their actions sometimes are used for propaganda purposes, substantive policy and technical criteria have slowly gained ground in this way. Thus, a stage is reached when practically all the candidates for public office have programs aimed at eradicating malnutrition and improving health conditions. In this sense, election periods are especially important.

As a general rule, to be successful as a planner, it is necessary to calculate not only the nutritional or health cost/benefit relationship of a given program but also the political costs and benefits. Only those professionals who, having calculated the nutritional cost/benefit ratio of a given program, then were able to translate that data into a political equation, have proven to be successful in getting their ideas implemented as policies and programs.

Another important consideration is to implement nutritional and health policies that last over time, beyond the term of the current government. Very frequently in Latin America new governments have a tendency to change what the previous ones have done. The success observed in Chile is due in great part to the fact that programs have been maintained and perfected through time. In this respect, our institute has also had an important role.[5] Every political system or government has its supporters and enemies; and programs, with their successes and failures, necessarily will come to be identified with the government in power. Professional planners responsible for these programs will, therefore, also come to be identified with a particular government.

The crucial point for the professional is to reach an acceptable balance between political involvement and independence. This is perhaps the key point: to keep the programs running beyond the term of the government in power. In this sense we have been in an exceptional position because our interventions have been carried out in a university setting and from the vantage point of a highly respected institution. It is essential to gain the confidence of the government in power and also of the community. The whole team of experts participating in a health and nutrition program have to be cautious not to get involved with contingent, changing, and short-lived issues. This is extremely difficult, especially in Latin American universities, because they can easily become instruments promoting a particular political point of view, despite the essential need to stay outside of the power struggle. Therefore, it is important for professionals to win support from all sides and to remain aloof from partisan political battles.

Finally, a nutritional and health policy has to be flexible, in the sense that it has to be adaptable to the socioeconomic strategy of the government. Planners try many times to do exactly the opposite: to adapt governmental socioeconomic policies to the needs of a nutrition and health policy. Lack of flexibility is unrealistic and underlies many failures. Policy has to be developed in such a way that it is compatible with different political philosophies and political realties, ranging from a socialist economic system to a liberal, market economy. This has been the case in

Chile, where nutritional and health policies have survived shifts from one extreme to the other. During the last thirty years, in spite of different governments and economic strategies, the basic principles behind health and nutrition have been maintained, while program efficiency and coverage have been improved. In addition, new interventions were implemented regardless of changing circumstances. This means that health and nutrition policies have to be flexible and should never be linked to any particular political group or ideology.

Health and Nutrition

In an underdeveloped country, a high percentage of people live in extremely impoverished conditions and are subject to high risk. They also are totally marginalized people, living outside the socioeconomic structures of society. Because of this, it is difficult to reach them with the basic services provided by the government. These people were born in extreme poverty and this condition has persisted for many generations. Furthermore, they do not anticipate any change in their lot. Nor do they perceive the benefits they could obtain from the services provided by the government. People living in extreme poverty lack the capacity to become organized, and they do not and cannot exert political pressure to obtain favorable legislation. Many governments have organized health systems for groups that can exert pressure such as blue- or white-collar workers, the military, and the middle class, while ignoring or paying little heed to marginal rural and urban groups.

From our point of view, the first step in a sound nutrition and health policy is to organize a national health infrastructure. This would cover the entire population, and especially the lower socioeconomic groups, and offer free services for those who cannot afford them. This has been the case in Chile: in 1952, several organizations that provided health care were merged and transformed into the National Health Service. Since then, preventive medicine has been provided free of charge to the entire population.

In the beginning, only a small percentage of the population was covered, but coverage has extended to the whole country, excluding only those who can afford private medical care. At present, the National Health Service has 35,000 hospital beds and 1,480 health clinics and health centers throughout the country. The National Health Service employs 58,000 persons, including 4,520 physicians, 1,365 dentists, 2,090 registered nurses, 1,690 midwives, 768 social workers, 710 nutritionists, and 24,480 nurses aides.

In the thirty years that the service has been in operation, coverage has been not only extended but also made more effective. The personnel have developed an attitude of service and commitment to the community, whose respect they have gained. In turn, the population has become aware of its rights and responsibilities in relation to health care. Thus, for example, examinations during pregnancy have increased considerably, 98 percent of births now take place in hospitals, and an estimated 95 percent of all children are regularly given immunizations. As a consequence, the incidence of diseases, such as measles and whooping cough, has declined considerably, and poliomyelitis and tetanus neonatorum have been eradicated. Regular check-ups of children have become routine and provide weight-for-age data for over 90 percent of the preschool children, who are evaluated every three months.

Family planning has been included among health activities since 1966 and has resulted in a considerable decrease in fertility. Currently, a large percentage of women are using contraceptives and this has contributed to the decline in population growth from an annual rate of 2.9 percent to the present rate 1.48 percent. The decrease has taken place mainly in the low socioeconomic groups. Because of this, a significant decrease in infant mortality and malnutrition has been observed. From 1962 to 1981, the crude birth rate decreased from thirty-eight to twenty-three per thousand, in particular among families with four or more children, where the greatest incidence of malnutrition is usually found. There also have been fewer births to women thirty-five years of age or older, a situation which has contributed to the decline in neonatal mortality. The decrease in the birth rate is responsible for 20 percent of the reduction in the infant mortality rate.[6]

From the beginning, a program of nutritional intervention was implemented through the National Health Service. It includes free distribution of powdered milk for every child up to two, and weaning foods for children between two and five. The program also includes powdered milk distribution to lactating and pregnant mothers (Table 5-2).

The food is distributed through the *primary health care centers* and this food distribution becomes a motivation for undertaking other health care activities. Food distribution had been extremely important not only from the nutritional point of view but also as a mechanism to attract mothers to the health care centers. To achieve these goals, the products distributed and their packaging and display have been of excellent quality. Special care has been taken to avoid the feeling that these programs are designed for poor people. The same products and services compete successfully in the open market.

The food distribution program started in 1951. In the beginning, the amount of milk dispensed was limited but increased gradually as the national health service developed. Figures 5-5 and 5-6 show that there exists a close relationship between the amount of food distributed and the number of visits to a primary health care facility. The linkage between attendance at health care centers and food distribution means that in the public mind both programs are interrelated and complementary.

In short, an efficient health care infrastructure and rational nutritional programs have been two basic factors that explain the dramatic decline in malnutrition and infant and preschool mortality in Chile between 1960 and 1974. The improvements during this period served as a foundation for progress later on. The implementation of the health system with its broad coverage has led not only to effective nutritional programs oriented at target groups but also to other interventions such as family planning, health controls, immunizations, health and nutrition education, and the promotion of breast-feeding. The fact that the community has developed a true "culture of health" and has awakened to the need to preserve it through the health service is of paramount importance.

Table 5-2

Amounts of Food Distributed Monthly by the National Health Service to Children and Mothers

Group	Product	Amount (kg per month)	Composition (per 100 gm)	
			Calories	Protein (gm)
Children				
0–5 months	Milk, 26% fat	3	496	27
6–23 months	Milk, 26% fat	2	496	27
2–5 years	Weaning food	1.5	420	20
Women				
Pregnant	Milk, 12% fat	2	410	31.6
Nursing	Milk, 26% fat	3	496	27

Source: N. González, A. Infante, L. Schlesinger, and F. Monckeberg, *Nutrition Intervention Strategies in National Development*, Barbara A. Underwood, ed. (New York: Academic Press, 1983), p. 103.

Note: In each instance, "milk" means powdered milk.

Our Experience in Nutritional Policy

Despite all of these advances, in 1974 malnutrition in Chile still affected 16 percent of the preschool children while infant and preschool mortality was 60 and 4 per thousand, respectively. A new strategy was, therefore, required and for this purpose the government created the Council for Food and Nutrition (Consejo Nacional para la Alimentación y Nutrición, CONPAN) in 1974. This was an autonomous, interministerial agency entrusted with the preparation and coordination of a nutritional policy for the country. The agency had a council composed of the ministers of health, economy, education, agriculture, work and social welfare,

Figure 5-5

Children Attended by the National Health Service and Amount of Milk Distributed

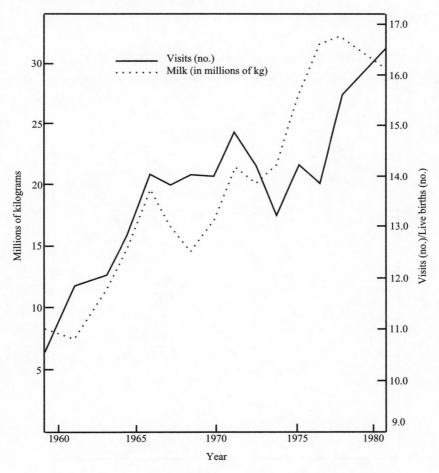

Source: N. Gonzalez, A. Infante, L. Schlesinger, and F. Monckeberg, "Effectiveness of Supplementary Feeding Programs in Chile," in *Nutrition Intervention Strategies in National Development,* ed. Barbara A. Underwood (New York: Academic Press, 1983), p. 103.

Note: As milk distribution increases, there is also an increased utilization of medical services.

and planning. CONPAN had an executive coordinator to supervise the technical and administrative coordination of the agency's activities, a position I had the privilege of serving in.

CONPAN resulted in a new nutrition policy with the aim of ensuring the best possible nutritional situation for the entire population within the limits of the country's resources. Special emphasis was placed on protecting the most vulnerable groups. The new policy encompassed the entire food chain and the concerns

Figure 5-6

Prenatal Visits and Amount of Food Distributed

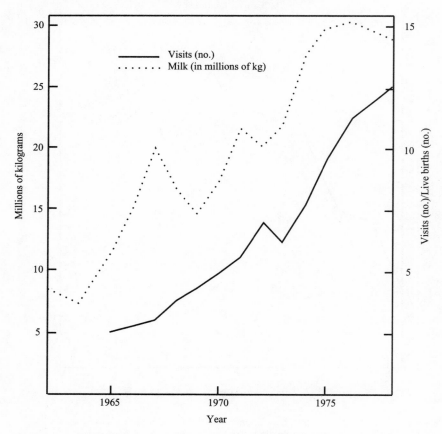

Source: N. Gonzalez, A. Infante, L. Schlesinger, and F. Monckeberg, "Effectiveness of Supplementary Feeding Programs in Chile," in *Nutrition Intervention Strategies in National Development,* ed. Barbara A. Underwood (New York: Academic Press, 1983), p. 103.

Note: As food distribution increases, so does the number of visits of pregnant women.

for food security, food production, imports, food marketing, income, quality control, nutrition education, micronutrient disorders, nutritional diseases, and sanitation.[7]

We soon realized that these concepts were absolutely theoretical. To articulate a nutrition policy is one thing; to try to implement it is a completely different situation. Numerous obstacles became apparent. Resources were limited; bureaucratic resistance surfaced; vested interests emerged; and, finally, rivalries among different ministers arose, reflecting the fact that few would accept interference in their own areas of responsibility. We learned the hard way than an ideal nutrition policy may be an impossible dream and that perhaps, after all, it may not be necessary. Therefore, we concentrated our efforts on specific interventions aimed at improving the nutritional condition of specific target groups.

CONPAN had a short life and was disbanded by a government decree. After that, we changed the strategy to establish direct relationships with particular ministers and with key people in the different sectors. This approach proved to be much more effective. Our conclusion was that one should not pretend to have a comprehensive nutrition policy or an official body to coordinate the interventions of the different sectors. Coordination and evaluation are extremely difficult tasks in any government. The essential points are to exert leadership, to have credibility based on scientific and technical authority, and to exhibit flexibility and, most of all, persistence and patience. Again, it should be noted, this has been the critical role played by the university and, more specifically, by INTA.

In retrospect, I think the rather brief existence of CONPAN was necessary. Methodologies for solving significant problems were developed and many of the interventions that were designed have been successfully implemented afterwards. Above all, the government became aware of the need for scientifically based programs that seek to help groups, that have been excluded from the economic and political structures of the country. After describing this experience, I have to say that in the end, considerable progress has been achieved during this last period, which I will attempt to summarize by sectors—health and nutrition, education, and agriculture.

Health and Nutrition Sector

A data collection system was developed, specifically targeted to the nutritional condition of children up to six. Every child under the care of the National Health Service (an estimated 1.35 million children) is measured every three months and his or her weight for age is calculated. Basic information is gathered about families, in order to examine socioeconomic conditions and related health risk factors. Information about weight at birth is collected regularly for all the deliveries in the hospitals of the country.

Food and Nutrition Interventions

Targeted food interventions for families in extreme poverty have been developed. For these groups, a food distribution program, including staples such as rice, wheat flower, and oil, was established through the primary health care centers. The objective of this program is to improve the nutrition of both the children and their families. Selected for this program are families of children with low birth weight (less than 2.5 kg); children whose weight increase has been inadequate for two months; and children born to mothers under twenty. Also participating are families with five or more children and families with severe socioeconomic problems.

Table 5-3

Clinical Progress of Marasmic Infants During Four Months of Treatment

	Admission	50 Day	100 Day	150 Day
Weight Deficit for Age (g)				
Group A	56 ± 8	54 ± 13	48 ± 12	40 ± 13
Group B	55 ± 5	36 ± 8	21 ± 6	16 ± 3
		$p<0.001$	$p<0.001$	$p<0.001$
Height Deficit for Age (cm)				
Group A	76 ± 10	70 ± 17	65 ± 16	65 ± 14
Group B	82 ± 13	50 ± 14	32 ± 6	21 ± 7
		$p<0.001$	$p<0.001$	$p<0.001$
Psychomotor Development Quotient				
Group A	56 ± 8	60 ± 11	64 ± 14	65 ± 12
Group B	55 ± 5	71 ± 10	80 ± 8	85 ± 1
		$p<0.01$	$p<0.001$	$p<0.001$

Source: F. Monckeberg, *Nutrition in the 1980s* (New York: Alan R. Liss, Inc., 1980), p. 141.

Notes: Group A consists of eighty infants treated in a conventional pediatric hospital. Group B consists of eighty infants treated in a CONIN center.

Treatment of Malnourished Children

Children suffering from severe malnutrition now have access to treatment. This program has had a direct influence on infant mortality. A 1974 study showed that approximately 8,200 children a year, on an average, became severely malnourished. A follow-up study confirmed that infants with severe malnutrition prior to six months of age, had an 85 percent chance of dying before they were one.[8] Analysis of cases of severe malnutrition showed that almost all occurred in children under two years of age, and 80 percent of the affected children were less than six months of age.

A pilot project was started in 1975 to tackle this program, with the aim of rehabilitating infants with severe malnutrition. For this purpose a specialized Nutritional Recovery Center was set up with forty beds for infants. Each malnourished infant remained as an inpatient until fully recovered; he or she was given appropriate food and underwent a program of cognitive, affective, and motor stimulation. The mother was involved in the treatment and received education and training. The results of this pilot study were impressive. No deaths occurred among the children in treatment, although inpatient mortality had previously been about 25 percent, and very satisfactory rehabilitation had been attained in both nutritional and psychomotor terms (Table 5-3 and Figure 5-7).

CONIN

In view of the success of the pilot project, INTA set up a private foundation, called the Chilean Nutrition Foundation (Corporacion para la Nutrición Infantil, CONIN), in order to extend the pilot program throughout the country. Within three years, with funds amounting to US$9 million provided by the community, thirty-three centers were built, equipped, and put into operation in different cities of the country. The installed capacity covers all needs, with 1,500 beds that make it possible to treat every year through full recovery 3,400 children with severe malnutrition.

Each center has forty to sixty beds, full medical facilities, a milk kitchen and a laundry, and the staff includes a full-time manager and six health professionals—a pediatrician, nutritionist, registered nurse, nursery teacher, and a social worker. Forty nurses aides work in three shifts, and eighty volunteers work on individual stimulation programs and follow-up at home. Operational costs are financed under an agreement with the National Health Service (which covers 80 percent of the costs) and partly by CONIN-raised funds.[9] The cost per day is US$6.50 per child and the total cost of rehabilitating one severely malnourished infant is US$600. CONIN has a staff of 1,400, along with 2,300 voluntary workers.

The program has had a notable impact in reducing the numbers of children suffering from severe malnutrition and in reducing the incidence of infant malnutrition. It is estimated that CONIN helps prevent almost two thousand deaths annually among infants under twelve months of age. In terms of overall infant mortality, this means that the program is responsible for over 20 percent of the reduction in infant mortality. During the years in which the program has been operational, over fifty thousand infants have been rehabilitated, with an average mortality rate of 2 percent. Follow-up studies show that 98 percent of the children who have recovered continue to have satisfactory weight gain at home, and only 1.8 percent have required readmission in a center.

CONIN has now embarked on a new program that rehabilitates low birth-weight babies before returning them to their mothers. Studies have shown that this is a high-risk group which contributes significantly to mortality during the first two months of life. Affected infants remain in a center for thirty days, during which time the mothers receive instruction on child care.

Breast-Feeding

Because a large share (85 percent) of Chile's population lives in urban areas and perhaps as a result of the system of free milk distribution, there has been an abrupt decline in the practice of breast-feeding. In 1940, 85 percent of the infants were breast-fed up to the age of six months. By 1967 this proportion had decreased to 25 percent, and by 1974 to 19 percent.[10] This decline undoubtedly contributed to the increase in early, severe malnutrition. Consequently, an extensive program was introduced to promote breast-feeding, using both the mass media (e.g., radio, television, magazines) and formal education. In particular, a firm stand was taken on this issue in the professional medical community and in the schools that train child health care workers such as midwives, nurses, and health educators. Professional and auxiliary personnel have received instruction provided by the National Health Service. Printed materials illustrating the importance of breast-feeding and how to advance it have been prepared and distributed.

As a consequence there has been a noticeable change of attitude in the population and among health care personnel, and breast-feeding has increased significantly. More than 52 percent of mothers now breast-feed their children during the first ninety days, representing an 80 percent increase in the first three months of life.[11]

Nutrition Education

A nutrition education program was created by CONPAN and included nutrition training at both the elementary and intermediate school levels. Textbooks have been prepared, although they have not been put in use. However, in the health sector, there has been considerable progress with nutrition training. It has been possible to staff each national health service clinic with a nutritionist who is responsible for implementing the nutrition education program. Nutritionists, who are required to undergo five years of university courses, have been carrying out important work in both the prevention and treatment of malnutrition.

Figure 5-7

Weight Increase in Seventy Severely Malnourished Infants after Four Months of Treatment

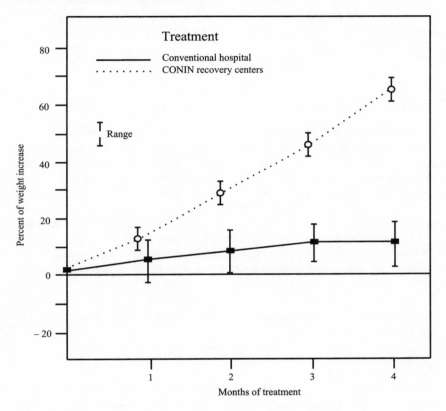

Source: F. Monckeberg and J. Riumallo, "Nutrition Recovery Centers: The Chilean Experience," in *Nutrition Intervention Strategies in National Development*, p. 189.

Rural Health Care

Because 85 percent of Chile's population is urban, the National Health Service has adequate coverage in urban areas, but it has been more difficult to provide coverage in rural areas, especially in the most isolated regions. Medical and nutritional care for rural communities is provided by health posts, each of which has a full-time health worker whose activities are complemented by regular visits of health teams. These health posts also provide nutrition programs.

In order to increase health care for pregnant rural women and provide adequate access to the nearest maternity facility, a program known as Hostels for

Rural Mothers was implemented. The idea was to build these accommodations near to maternity hospitals and to allow pregnant women from rural areas to stay there during the fifteen days prior to, as well as up to ten days after, the delivery. The women also receive instruction from hospital staff concerning nutrition, breast-feeding, and child care. Sixty-four of these hostels have been set up in conjunction with maternity hospitals in primary health care areas. Along with other measures they have significantly decreased neonatal mortality by reducing the risks inherent in delivery.

Educational Sector

During the past thirty years a considerable improvement has occurred in elementary education. In 1960, more than 30 percent of the population was illiterate, while at present less than 4 percent is in this condition. Only 10 percent of the children in 1960 had completed elementary education. Today, 85 percent of the children complete eight years of elementary education.

It is particularly important to draw attention to the emphasis that has been placed on education for mothers, as this has a strong bearing on malnutrition and infant mortality. The latter is five times higher among mothers who have not completed elementary education than among those who have completed it.[12] Progress in the educational field is particularly noticeable among women who were illiterate during their child-bearing years. This figure fell to 6 percent by 1982. In the period 1969–82, there was a noticeable decrease in the number of births to women with a low level of education (i.e., either without education or with only elementary-level education).

School Food Programs

The school feeding program, although technically not a nutritional intervention program since it only can provide limited daily calories and proteins required, has had a very important effect in reducing school desertion. CONPAN reviewed the program, reaching the conclusion that its implementation should be transferred to private agencies that could provide the complete service and leaving to the Ministry of Education the role of evaluation and control. This reorganization improved the quality of the service, and accomplished the goal of combating school desertion. At present, the program during 180 days of the school year supplies 750,000 breakfasts and 550,000 lunches daily to 4,000 schools across the country.

Preschool Food Programs

The largest proportion of malnourished children in Chile live in deprived urban areas, as a consequence of the massive migration to the cities that took place during the last decade. Almost every city has a belt of shantytowns surrounding it. Experience shows that it is difficult to prevent malnutrition in children from population groups with a low socioeconomic and educational level, even when free food is provided. Moreover, a number of studies indicate that extreme poverty causes damage to the physical and intellectual capabilities of individuals. This damage is the result not only of malnutrition, but of other factors inherent in chronic poverty.

Against this background, CONPAN supported the development of a day care center program for preschool children living in extreme urban poverty. Children attend the centers during the day, where all their food is provided and where they also undergo psychomotor and affective stimulation. During the last ten years, 850 such centers have been built and equipped, covering 110,000 preschool children between two and six. According to earlier estimates by CONPAN, the program will eventually cover 160,000 children, which is the number believed to be at risk of malnutrition and living in extreme poverty in urban areas.[13]

Homeless Children

A program for homeless and troubled children is designed to provide care in live-in centers for children from two to twelve years of age. These children include orphans, abandoned children, and children who display maladjusted behavior. The aim is to restore the child to a normal behavioral situation, combat child vagrancy, and improve the conditions of life. The program has been extended and improved through the building of new centers and now covers 39,000 children.

Sanitation Sector

Overcrowding and inadequate sanitation in urban areas are common to all Latin American countries. This situation has become worse in the past few decades as a result of the explosive growth of the population and increased migration to the cities. In 1974, a high percentage of the population in Chile lived in extremely impoverished areas that lacked sanitation facilities. Inadequate sanitation adversely affects child nutrition and gives rise to gastrointestinal and other infectious diseases. Diluted, contaminated infant formulas are one of the main contributors to the shift in the incidence of malnutrition to the early months of life and this, in turn, is associated with high risk of death.

For these reasons, CONPAN developed a program that emphasized the importance of sanitation in preventing early malnutrition. During the initial stage of this program, a brick-and-timber sanitary unit was built on the plots of three hundred families living in a slum area. Each unit had a kitchen and a bathroom and an outdoor sink for washing clothes. The kitchen was equipped with shelves, and a sink; the bathroom had a lavatory, flush toilet, and shower. Hot water also was supplied. The unit was connected to the general sewerage system.[14]

The results demonstrated a significant causal link between environmental sanitation and improvements in both nutrition and the quality of life. Perhaps the most significant result was the striking change in the attitudes of the families. The pessimistic and fatalistic approach to life, the hopelessness and acceptance of the miserable life prevailing in the community before the sanitary unit was installed, had changed into a sincere and deeply felt desire for improvement in their living conditions. This resulted in increased individual efforts and in motivation to meet the challenge of improving the quality of life.

These results led to the development of a nationwide sanitation program to improve the sanitary situation of the urban population. In the past ten years 220,000 sanitary units have been built in different cities of the country. In 1960, only 40 percent of the population had drinking water in their homes, and only 35 percent had an adequate sewerage system. At present, 98 percent of the population have drinking water at home, and 79 percent live in housing connected to a sewerage system (Figure 5-8). There is no doubt that improved sanitary conditions have also been important factors in the decrease in malnutrition and in the improvements in health conditions.

Agriculture Sector

Agriculture and food production are fundamental elements in any nation's development process and a precondition to raising the state of health and nutrition among people. As I have emphasized earlier, the economic development of Chile as expressed in per capita GNP, for the most part, has not been very considerable during the last forty years. From the beginning of the present century, the Chilean economy was based primarily on the export of raw materials: first, nitrates, and later, copper. Industrial development started only after World War II, but this development was based on import substitution, with a high degree of protectionism. Agricultural development was retarded, because of artificially fixed prices, the high cost of imported commodities, and the lack of incentives. As a consequence, agricultural production increased less than population growth, and the failure of agricultural production to keep pace resulted in the ever-increasing importation of food.

In 1970, a socialist government was elected and an agrarian reform was implemented. This reform resulted in the expropriation of more than 60 percent of the total land under cultivation in the country. Agricultural production came almost totally under government control. A year later, agricultural production had nearly collapsed, and enormous amounts of food, equivalent to 70 percent of all the requirements, had to be imported.[15]

Three years later, in 1973, a military coup defeated the socialist government, and a free and open market economy was created. In 1974, CONPAN and the Ministry of Agriculture established a new agricultural policy, based on the following principles: 1) transfer of state-owned land to peasants and farmers; 2) free-market prices for every agricultural product and the elimination of all state subsidies; 3) guaranteed prices for basic products; 4) technology transfer to farmers; 5) construction of an irrigation infrastructure; and, 6) a new credit policy.

Figure 5-8

Urban Coverage of Potable Water and Sewerage Services, 1976–1987

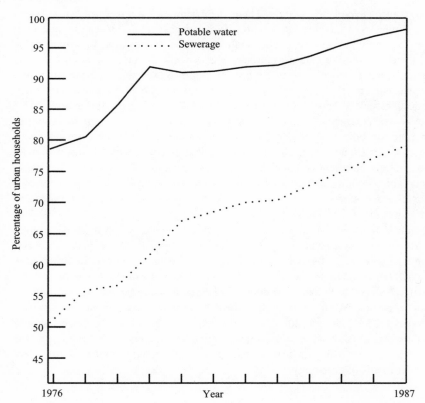

Source: Informe Anual (Santiago, Chile: Ministry of Public Works, National Service of Sanitary Works, 1988), p. 18.

Note: Includes both in-house connections and access to water from a nearby source.

As a result of these changes, a rapid increase in agricultural production was achieved, with an annual growth rate of 7 percent, during the last ten years. The value of food imports fell from US$700 million in 1973 to US$80 million annually at present. In the last eight years a remarkably strong agricultural sector, consisting of fruit and vegetable production and agroindustrial development, has been established. Today, this has become one of the most dynamic economic sectors, which in 1988 accounted for US$1,637 million per year in exports. The success of Chile's agricultural sector has led not only to a sharp decline in costly food imports but also to a substantial increase in rural employment and income and, correspondingly, to a marked improvement in health and nutrition.

Summary

The Chilean experience, presented here, demonstrates that it is possible to successfully implement targeted interventions in health, sanitation, education, and food production that lead to substantial improvements in the health and nutrition status of the population, despite the persistence of poverty and underdevelopment. This result is important because it has been possible to prevent to a large extent the physical and psychological injury of large numbers of Chile's infants and children. Negative societal and environmental factors, by hindering the full expression of the genetic potential of the population, work to impede development. We consider that the capabilities of the population constitute the most precious asset any country has. If we want to reach satisfactory levels of development, this resource must be carefully protected and nurtured. Our experience may be useful to other countries with whom we share similar problems. Of course, the successful utilization of our experience requires an analysis of local realities and the adaptation of the programs to these realities.

It is important to emphasize that the process described in these pages took place over several decades. Its success was due mainly to the persistence and continuity of programs over time and to continued improvements in their implementation. In the future, periodic adaptation of programs to the prevailing circumstances, along with sound economic strategies to improve the situation of the poorer groups, will have to be implemented in order to consolidate the advances already made. If these conditions are not met, these gains may be lost because in reality they already exceed the economic limits of the country, that is, what might be expected given the limited economic growth and limited income that are evident in many parts of the county.

Notes

1.   F. Monckeberg, S. Valiente, and F. Mardones, "Infant and Preschool Nutrition: Economical Development Versus Intervention Strategies, The Case of Chile," *Nutrition Research* 7 (1987):327.

2.   F. Monckeberg, "The Possibilities for Nutrition Intervention in Latin America," *Food Technology* 35 (1981):115–21.

3.   Commission on Health Research Development, *Health Research: Essential Link to Equity in Development* (New York: Oxford University Press, 1990), 10.

4.   J. P. Terra, "Situación de la Infancia en Latinamérica y el Caribe." Remarks at the Annual Meeting of UNICEF, Mexico City, 16–18 May, 1979.

5.   F. Monckeberg, "Socioeconomic Development and Nutritional Status: Efficiency of Intervention Programs," in *Nutrition Intervention Strategies in National Development,* ed. Barbara A. Underwood (New York: Academic Press, 1983), 31.

6.   E. Taucher, "Effects of Declining Fertility on Infant Mortality Levels." New York: Rockefeller Foundation, 1986. Unpublished Report.

7.   F. Monckeberg, and Sergio Valiente, eds., *Food and Nutrition Policy in Chile*. (Santiago: Instituto de Nutrición y Tecnologia des los Alimentos, 1976).

8.   F. Monckeberg, and J. Riumallo, "Nutrition Recovery Centers: The Chilean Experience," in *Nutrition Intervention Strategies in National Development*, p. 189.

9.   Monckeberg and Riumallo, p. 189.

10.   F. Monckeberg, "Treatment of Severe Malnutrition During the First Year of Life," in *Nutrition in the 1980s: Constraints on Our Knowledge*, (New York: Alan R. Liss Inc., 1981), 141.

11.   N. Gonzalez et al., "Evaluación Preliminar del Programa de Fomento a la Lactancia Materna." *Review of Chilean Pediatrics* 54(1982):360.

12.   S. Valiente et al., Evolución de la Mortalidad Infantil y otrso Indicadores Conexos en Chile, entre 1962 y 1981. Unpublished Report.

13.   Monckeberg and Valiente.

14.   L. Schlesinger et al., "Environmental Sanitation: A Nutrition Intervention," in *Nutrition Intervention Strategies in National Development*, p. 241.

15.   F. Monckeberg, *Crear para Compartir y Comparatir para Seguir Creando* (Santiago: Editorial Andres Bello, 1980).

CHAPTER 6

Changing Health and Nutrition Behavior: A Social Marketing View

Eduardo L. Roberto
Coca-Cola Foundation Professor of International Marketing
Asian Institute of Management
Manila, the Philippines

Nearly two decades ago, the Brookings Institution and the Foundation for Child Development commissioned Alan Berg to study the role of nutrition in national development. In the conclusion of his study, Berg said: "Knowledge of nutrition—the problems as well as the techniques and technologies to meet them—is at a stage where much can be done. Enough information already is in hand to justify resource allocations for nutrition on a substantial scale."[1] At a 1988 Smithsonian Institution colloquium on world food issues, John Mellor echoed Berg and said that what we already know regarding the nutrition problem "is now ample and sound."[2]

In the same colloquium, Gelia Castillo asked: "Why, why haven't we done more—when the problem seems to be well defined, the solutions well researched, and the actions required seem to be so obviously doable?"[3] Dutra de Oliveira gave a simple answer: "We have to try to apply what we know."[4] It is the doing that counts. However, merely shifting the focus of our attention from planning to implementing, and appreciating implementation's critical importance in getting results, does not mean that things will be done or done right. Knowing what is doable does not necessarily mean it will be done. Knowing what is actionable does not mean it will be acted upon. What will make a difference is actually taking action, something that Berg himself at the start of the seventies underscored: "If governments deem it important to eradicate major nutritional deficiencies, they must take actions."[5]

The key is to actually start doing the doable, to start implementing. But it should not be any kind of implementing. It should be the productive kind. In the 1988 Smithsonian colloquium, Berg recognized this and said: "Our policy understanding of what to do is in most places far ahead of our understanding of how to do it. There are many good policies in place. There are many good programs in place. . . . But implementation is often appalling."[6]

I represent a practice and a discipline of implementation. It is a management practice called *social marketing*. This paper describes what this practice has learned about implementing nutrition and health programs. In the process, it illustrates what social marketing can do to answer Castillo's question and Berg's 1988 call for good implementation.

Focusing on implementation does not mean that research, appropriate technology, planning, and policy are less important. They are vitally important. Each forms a segment or part of an integral program management chain. Unfortunately, implementation in the past has been taken for granted. Development experts and social program planners are not to blame. The management discipline itself has taken implementation for granted. One has only to compare the planning and the control literature with the implementation literature to realize this. It was not until the Peters and Waterman study—showing that it is the superior implementing skills, the "hands-on management style," which differentiated the best-run from the mediocre companies—that implementation became as serious a concern for both management research and training as planning and control.[7]

Implementation is just as difficult a process and a skill as research, technology development, and planning and policy formulation. Its role in social program management is to supplement and to realize the values derived from these other tasks. After all, the fruits of research and technology cannot be enjoyed, and the objectives of planning and policy cannot be achieved, unless implementation has effectively brought the activities to the target population.

To implement a nutrition program means to put it into effect among a particular target population. Implementation's effects consist of bringing about specific nutrition behaviors and responses from the target population. Social marketing is about how those behaviors and responses may be effectively shaped.

Social Marketing and Health and Nutrition Intervention

Social marketing implements a nutrition program, or intervention, by taking these steps:

1. Identify the *target adopter segments* (i.e., the particular segments of, or groups in, the population among which behavior changes are sought after), assess their needs, and then assign a priority to the subgroups, or segments;

2. For each target segment, specify the behavioral responses to effect, or bring about, and for each response, determine the social marketing tool or set of tools needed to influence the behavior;

3. Integrate the identified social marketing tools into a comprehensive, coherent, and synergistic mix, and then field, or implement, this mix toward the goal of persuading a target population to adopt a desired set of behaviors. This is

accomplished through implementing a set of the appropriate tasks and managing personnel, procedures, controls, and an evaluation system.

A brief explanation of a few terms and concepts can be useful at this point. In any social intervention, target adopter segments refer to the groups of people who are the program's intended recipients and beneficiaries, or whose behavior the program is seeking to change or sustain. For example, Thailand's first National Food and Nutrition Plan targeted "the most vulnerable groups . . . because resources were limited." The plan identified four of them: 1) children five years of age or under, 2) school-age children, 3) pregnant women, and 4) lactating women.[8] These are examples of target adopter segments.

Nutrition programs that are focused on target adopter segments are different from other programs that utilize a development planning approach with a populationwide orientation. Studies have shown that target-segment-oriented programs are more cost-effective than populationwide ones.[9] But cost-effectiveness may not be the major consideration for developing nutrition interventions.[10]

A nutrition program, or intervention, formulated in a social marketing campaign will specify three target adopter responses. These are *target thoughts, target feelings,* and *target actions.* An element in a Papua, New Guinea, breast-feeding campaign was a law "making infant feeding bottles and nipples available only upon prescription from a registered health worker." The objective was to focus "the community's attention on the dangers of bottle-feeding without adequate safeguards," and to raise public "awareness of the problem."[11] This is an example of a target thought. A bread fortification program in India and its accompanying nutrition education campaign provide an example of a target feeling. Instead of appealing to its audience with a conventional nutritional message, the campaign communicated a "mothers who care" message, one emphasizing emotion and affect.[12] An Indonesian nutrition education program provides a number of examples of target actions. For instance, for the adopter segment of "mothers of infants from five to eight months," the program established three "distinct behavioral objectives: (1) breast-feed, using both breasts; (2) feed *bubur campur* (enriched rice porridge) four times a day; and (3) introduce the supplementary food patiently."[13]

Social marketing tools consist of what the literature refers to mnemonically as "the four P's," namely:

1. *Product,* or set of tools covering the physical as well as the perceived aspects of a program's intended effect or desired behavioral response, (e.g., a tangible product such as infant formula, its brand and packaging, that facilitates the achievement of the intended effect);

2. *Place,* or the set of tools for making the product available and accessible (also referred to as *distribution channels* and *service outlets*);

3. *Promotion,* or the set of tools used for informing, persuading, and moving the target adopter segments to adopt an idea or behavior now and not to postpone it

(this can include both mass, specialized, and direct response advertising, field extension work, and adoption promotion campaigns);

4. *Price,* or the set of tools used to make the cost of adopting the product affordable to the target adopter segments, both monetarily and nonmonetarily.

Segmenting and Assessing Needs

Health and nutrition programs addressing specific adopter groups such as pregnant women, lactating women, mothers of children with diarrhea, mothers of infants four months old or less, and so on, are clearly candidates for a segmentation strategy. But even nutrition programs aimed at the general public, such as a mass-media-based nutrition education campaign, find that in their program implementation it is cost-effective to segment.

Table 6-1

Assessing Target Adopter Needs at Successive Stages of Adoption

Selected Adoption Stages	Example: Adoption of Condom	Needs Assessment Technique(s)
Predisposition stage: Attitude formation	Attitude toward family planning: "I believe in family planning because it's the only way to protect my wife's health while at the same time attending to our sex life without risking pregnancy."	Focus group discussion (FGD) research plus attitude survey.
Decision stage: Choosing among alternative means	Choice of condom: "She had all the burden of pregnancy. Now, it's my turn to do something about preventing it. It's the best way to express my love for my wife."	FGD research plus family planning methods perceptions survey.
Usage/consumption stage: Use of the chosen means	Step-by-step use of the condom: "This is the way I use a condom. First, I . . ."	Step-by-step usage research.

Source: generated by author.

Segmenting a target population of adopters recognizes a practical reality. Not everyone has the same needs or behaves in the same way in relation to health and nutrition. Implementing a nutrition program has to start with identifying discrete segments that have similar needs and behaviors among them but that differ from the needs and behaviors of other population segments. Speedier adoptions can be attained by tailoring a program activity or intervention to fit each segment. This is what makes segmenting an economical implementation tool.

Setting priorities among the various segments is a management responsibility and decision. The task must reflect the nutrition program's mission. For instance, a program that pledges to reach the "poorest of the poor" has its top priority segment explicitly designated. In the absence of a program mission that makes explicit its target segment preferences, program management must exercise judgment about such preferences.

Following the selection of target segments comes the task of assessing segment needs. Social marketing has contributed to a better understanding of this task. It has extended needs assessment techniques by identifying needs across the entire range of the adoption process. An adopter segment's needs differ at different stages in the process. To ensure that nutrition program implementation is truly responsive, the needs of the target population at every stage of adoption should be determined and served. Table 6-1 illustrates this needs assessment approach in the specific case of a family planning program in the Philippines that seeks to promote the use of condoms for birth control.

Table 6-1 abbreviates for illustration purposes the adoption stages into three. At the predisposition stage, the needs assessment techniques of focus group discussion research, plus an attitude survey, determined the target adopter's primary family planning needs as the twin concerns for the wife's health and a sex life free from pregnancy risk. In the next stage of choosing a particular family planning method, the needs assessment techniques of focus group discussion research, plus a perception survey, found that for the condom, the target segment's immediate motivation was the need to assume responsibility for avoiding pregnancy. Finally, in the last stage of actually using the condom, the needs assessment method of step-by-step usage research indicated a whole new set of target segment needs. The research summary clarifies what those newly discovered needs are. In the Metro Manila area, the research found the following:

The typical Metro Manila condom user is essentially a planner. Before sex, he inspects the condom by unrolling it. Inspection is to check for any "factory defect." The user inspects by taking the following steps. First, he goes to the bathroom faucet and fills the unrolled condom with water. Then, while holding and closing the open end with the fingers of his left hand, he squeezes from below the water-filled condom. He does this with the thumb and forefinger of his right hand. He says: "If no water squirts out, then there's no factory defect."

After this, the condom needs rerolling for later use. Because the condom is wet, the user finds rerolling difficult. It needs drying first. Most use Johnson's Baby Powder for this. Once rerolled, the user notices that the condom now lacks lubrication. So he lubricates it. Most use Johnson's Baby Oil. Then, the condom is finally ready for use.

From these results, the program managers recognized that if a condom is to function as an effective contraceptive, a priority need of target adopters is for correct product knowledge. Condom users obviously did not know that the condoms already had a powdery, silicon-based lubrication. In fact, the use of other kinds of lubrication, such as Johnson's Baby Oil, can corrode the rubber of the condom. Therefore, the lack of product information can lead to degrading a condom's contraceptive effectiveness.

Outside Metro Manila, the step-by-step usage study found a different set of target segment needs at the usage level:

In the provincial and rural areas, the condom user's typical physical setting is important to appreciate. He is living in a one-room house. That room is the family's living room, dining room, and bedroom. The evening is usually pitch dark unless it is full moon. There was only 11% electrification of the countryside.

The condom user is essentially an impulsive user. Condom usage proceeds along the following steps. As he nears his climax, the condom user pulls out and looks for his condom. Right after withdrawal, he says: "Every second counts." In the darkness, his hands grope around the floor (as there typically were no beds and everyone slept on the floor) where he recalls placing the condom. Once he finds it, he quickly tears the plastic wrap and pulls out the condom. At times and in his haste, the condom slips from his fingers. When he is unable to immediately locate where it dropped, he forgets about the condom and goes right back to where he pulled out seven or eight seconds ago.

The program managers soon realized from these results that the target segment needed another type of condom if the adopters were to have effective contraception. The need was for a condom that could be located easily in the dark. This led the program donor to find a new supplier that within a few months produced a new type of condom: a luminous type that even on the darkest night a user could readily locate.

In Indonesia, needs assessment research for a breast-feeding nutrition program led to similar practical findings of adopter needs. In narrating how they actually undertook breast-feeding, women in Central Java indicated that they did so primarily with their left breast. They did this because they believed the left breast contained food and the right one was for the water. In breast-feeding her baby, the mother brings the baby to the left breast for the food. According to the research, "if the child seemed content, the water (in the right breast) was never proffered."[14] Tracing the steps in breast-feeding highlighted the need to correct adopter's misperceptions. Her right and left breasts were both usable and necessary for infant feeding.

A third example comes from a Philippine Ministry of Health program to disseminate oral rehydration solutions for use by rural mothers in coping with their diarrheal babies. At that time, in 1983, the oral rehydration therapy utilized an

79

ORESOL package that had two separate packets, one containing the sodium and the other, the glucose. The instructions on the packet ask the mother to pour and dissolve the content of both portions in a liter of water, and then to administer the solution to the sick infant. To find out how rural mothers actually used the product, several of them were given ORESOL packets to use for their babies in case of diarrhea. When later interviewed, some of the mothers frankly observed that the one-liter solution mix was "impractical." One explained that her baby just could not finish all the contents in a single day. This mother was reacting to the packet's instruction saying that once mixed, the solution had to be consumed "over a 6–12 hour period for infants, and over a 3–4 hour period for children." Beyond these periods, mothers were told that the solution was no longer drinkable. The packet instruction cautioned: "Administer only newly mixed solutions. Do not use left-overs." Midwives and health workers who distributed the ORESOL packets told mothers to discard whatever was left over. The mothers, however, found this idea alien to their cultural habit of never throwing away leftover food.

There were other rural mothers who said they were unable to use the product. When they explained this, the program staff discovered it had overlooked something extremely basic. These mothers did not own nor could they find a one-liter container. A few other mothers used only one side of the packet, the portion containing the sodium. They explained their behavior as follows. They did not know either what "sodium" or "glucose" meant. Second, they tried one packet containing the glucose portion and they regarded it as "quality sugar." So they proceeded to save the glucose from all the packets they received and store it in a jar, and use this quality sugar for "serving to guests for their coffee."

These examples should alert nutrition program planners to the necessity of extending the needs assessment task to all stages in the adoption process. If that task had not been so extended in the above cases, it is unlikely that the managers would have acquired practical knowledge of adopter needs, the knowledge that leads target populations to take the actions that are sought after.

Nutrition Behavior and Social Marketing

Having identified the needs of the program's target adopter segments, program implementers must now find the means of satisfying those needs (i.e., fulfilling adopter needs in ways that achieve the program goals). To accomplish this, the target segments have to be persuaded and influenced to behave in the desired way. Social marketing assumes that marketing variables under the implementer's control cause and can change target adopter behaviors. It views adopter behavior as falling under two categories: ultimate and intermediate. The ultimate behavior is continued and committed adoption of a set of behaviors that a program seeks to achieve in the target adopters. The intermediate category consists of the several intermediate and related behavioral responses that together over time lead to adoption. All the intermediate behaviors prepare the way for the ultimate committed adopter behavior.

Social Marketing Mix

According to the social marketing model, a committed adoption is a function of the entire social marketing mix. It does not come from one or two or three of its elements but from all of them together. Each of the intermediate adopter responses, however, will likely be a function of a specific social marketing mix element. For example, the response of an adopter in becoming aware of a nutrition "product" is a function of the marketing mix element of advertising. The response of an adopter in gaining access to a nutrition product is a function of the marketing element of distribution channels and service outlets. The adopter response of trying out a nutrition product without delay is a function of the mix element of adoption promotion. Table 6-2 identifies all such intermediate responses, including the ultimate, committed behaviors, and designates the social marketing mix element that helps to determine each response.

The social marketing mix is, therefore, a model of adopter behavior and responses. It is a theory of behavior, if theory and model are regarded as synonymous.[15] What kind of adopter behavior model does the social marketing mix offer? The model has at least three distinguishing characteristics. First, it advocates hounding the adopter until he or she changes to the desired behavior. The social marketing mix model prescribes that for a nutrition program to successfully bring target adopters to committed adoption, the intervention must pursue them relentlesslyùas they are watching, reading, listening, thinking, feeling, desiring, intending, trying, and deciding to continue or to drop out. When the nutrition intervention makes its presence felt in each and every one of these adopter responses, the target adopters will eventually and finally accede to the program goals. They will adopt the desired behaviors and continue to do so for as long as a nutrition program effectively satisfies their nutrition and health needs.

This model of persistently affecting behavior changes is also a thorough model; thoroughness is its second characteristic. It works with virtually all of the known controllable determinants of behavior. A number of them have been popular in social and economic development programs in the past. For example, a major determinant is mass communication, which in social marketing is known as advertising. This variable held fascination for social planners in the 1940s and the 1950s. Another is the incentives variable, the social marketing mix element known as adoption promotion. Behavior modification advocates popularized this element in population control, health, and nutrition programs. Yet another came to be known as the "basic needs" approach, which emphasized something called a "needs satisfaction variable." This corresponds to the social marketing mix element of social product design and positioning. The U.S. Agency for International

Development championed this approach in its Third World assistance programs during the 1970s.

Table 6-2

Target Adopter Behaviors and Responses and Relevant Social Marketing Tools

Sequence of Target Adopter Behaviors and Responses	Social Marketing Tool(s)
Get adopters quickly informed and persuaded in great numbers.	Advertising.
Get them to implement their persuasion now and not later.	Adoption promotion.
Get them to avail themselves of the social product and have a satisfactory service delivery experience at the service outlets.	Distribution, placement, and service delivery.
Get them to be able to afford the social product both monetarily and nonmonetarily.	Adoption costs management and pricing.
Get them in a trial adoption of the product.	Social marketing mix.
Get them to be satisfied with their product adoption experience.	Social product quality.
Get them into retrial and committed adoption.	Social marketing mix.

Source: generated by the author.

The social marketing mix model advances at least two basic propositions about these variables. First, each of them is important to consider in influencing adopter behavior. Second and more importantly, each alone is not enough to affect the ultimate adopter behavior. For instance, mass communication is not enough because, as Table 6-2 shows, it can address only one of the series of necessary adopter responses leading to the ultimate adopter behavior.

A third critical characteristic of the model is that the social marketing mix combines its elements in ways to foster synergy. The marketing mix elements of product design, positioning, advertising, pricing, distribution, field and outreach, adoption promotion, and service delivery are placed together to explicitly ensure and facilitate interdependence. In this manner, they mutually reinforce one another. This makes the impact of the mix greater than the sum of the individual effects. Like the other characteristics, this does not arise automatically. The program implementer must purposefully and creatively engineer a synergistic whole.

When applied with its relentless, thorough, and synergistic characteristics, social marketing has demonstrated its effectiveness in changing adopter behavior. This positive side of social marketing has not been without its negative. Precisely because of its relentless pursuit of target adopter responses and the thoroughness and synergy of its efforts, social marketing has been labeled as manipulative. Often, the approach is feared precisely because it can work so successfully.

Starting with Product Analysis

How then is a social marketing mix actually implemented? With regard to health and nutrition intervention, the task starts with a focus on the last intermediate adopter response, as listed in Table 6-2. This involves adopter satisfaction with a product or service. A social marketing intervention has as its objective the adoption by a target population of a particular action, practice, or behavior. This would include adoption of a tangible product, such as an oral rehydration kit, or use of a social service, or committing an action (e.g., taking an infant to a clinic for a health check-up). Table 6-3 describes the range of adopter responses.

Achieving an adopter satisfaction response requires the program implementer to answer two questions:

1. Is the intervention's product capable of satisfying the pertinent needs of the target adopter segments?
2. Is it going to satisfy adopter needs better than other available products or better than before?

A "no" to the first question means that the nutrition program does not as yet have an effective product. It should, therefore, abort implementation at this point, and start over again with its product development or, in this case, redevelopment. A "yes" means that the product or service to be marketed is likely to be effective at least 50 percent of the time. The program implementer then has to focus on the second question.

Working on the second question will end up with any one of three alternative answers:

1. Yes, this is better.
2. No, it is just as good as the others or as before.
3. No, it is not better; it is less satisfying.

The first answer means that the nutrition program has a superior product; the second answer, it has a parity product (i.e., a product that lacks a competitive advantage over other products); and the third case, an inferior product.

A health and nutrition program with a superior product has a solid base from which to attain its target adopter behavior. Under such circumstances, the program will make less exacting demands on the other social marketing mix elements in order to attain the adopter behavioral objective. However, this will not be the case with a parity product. To pull the adopters into the program, the other social marketing mix elements must make up for what the parity product lacks in perceived superiority. The most demanding case is an inferior product. Advertising, distribution, field and outreach, pricing, adoption promotion, and service delivery all must then be enlisted to make up for the product's shortcomings. If a nutrition program implementer is faced with an inferior product for adoption, why then does the implementer still talk of going through with the process? Why not abort it?

Table 6-3

Range of Differences in Using Marketing in Health and Nutrition Programs

Range of Social Products	Examples	Closeness to Business Marketing	Applicability of Marketing
Tangible products	Oral rehydration solution; contraceptives, such as condoms	Very close	Relatively easy to apply the familiar, conventional marketing framework
Intangible products	Breast-feeding practice; birth control practice	Very far	Difficult (i.e., requiring a modified or new framework)

Source: generated by the author.

Implementations are necessarily situational. Consider the case of a calamity or the situation in which a program aims to reach a remote, inaccessible area in which the overriding consideration is simply the timely availability of a life-saving or life-giving product or service. In these situations, even an inferior product becomes acceptable. It is in those other situations, where time and resources allow for consideration of alternatives to satisfy adopters, that rejection of inferior products becomes feasible.

After analyzing the product's need-satisfying status, implementation proceeds to the task of effectively bringing the product to the target adopter segments for a committed adoption. This adoption will happen only if the program implementers and target adopters accomplish the following tasks:

1. Make the product or service available to the target adopters and give them access to it through distribution channels and service outlets, providing high quality and satisfying service;

2. Inform and persuade quickly and in great numbers the target adopter segments through the use of mass advertising;

3. Follow through this mass informing and persuasion with direct nonpersonal as well as personal communication efforts via media and through field and extension work;

4. Get the target adopters to adopt immediately and not later by means of its adoption promotion program;

5. Get the target adopters to continue adopting, and not to drop out, by means of its participatory promotion efforts;

6. Make affordable the product or service both monetarily and nonmonetarily, chiefly by means of pricing.

Task 1 constitutes the placement function of the four P's, mentioned earlier. Tasks 2 to 5 make up the promotion functions, and Task 6, pricing. What then has been learned in applying these marketing functions, which normally operate in business, to social programs and the field of nutrition and health interventions?

Product Availability and Service Outlets

Some social programs implementers in tackling the placement function have sought to utilize the business sector's distribution and selling capabilities. They find, however, that the available placement channels are not necessarily set up for social and development priorities. The Philippine Ministry of Health's campaign for ORESOL, for example, and the Population Commission's family planning program encountered this obstacle.

For the oral rehydration program, the government thought that channeling ORESOL through the more than two hundred thousand store outlets all over the country would be much more effective than using the Ministry's three thousand health centers. The superior number, however, concealed the reality that the business sector's distribution capabilities did not reach remote areas where the neediest target population segments resided. Furthermore, the commercial distributors were volume traders. They concentrated their network in areas where there was a profitable and *effective demand*, or market size, which consists of the total number of people multiplied by their purchasing power and then multiplied by usage or consumption frequency. In commercial terms, areas that have a large number of people but low disposable income are rated as low-priority areas. Yet for the ORESOL campaign, these were precisely the areas with the most unmet needs and, therefore, that deserved top priority.

This is not to say that the Philippine public health sector with its three thousand health centers was better set up for the oral rehydration campaign. A study of the Philippine rural health delivery system found that "none of the programs serve the poor groups to a greater extent than the rich."[16] If this is true of the national health structure, then the public sector is in no better shape than the business sector. But this is not the issue.

Placement is not only a matter of quantity or number of well-located service outlets, but also a matter of quality. *Quality placement* measures what the adopters will find in the service outlets. The outlets serve as points of consumption of goods and services and, therefore, of adopter satisfaction or the lack thereof. Health and nutrition service delivery programs that utilize a market-driven approach are more likely to achieve adopter satisfaction. One particular marketing approach that has proven to be effective is to treat service delivery functions as if they were dramatic roles, as in theater plays. Giving target adopters a satisfying experience then would depend upon combining the three essential elements of a good play: *actors,* or the service personnel; the *stage,* or the service outlet ambiance; and the *staging,* or the service performance itself. All three must be well managed. When they are, the outcome is a satisfied adopter who is motivated to spread the good news to others and to help multiply the adoptions elsewhere. When they are poorly executed, the results are disastrous.[17]

A family planning program targeted to promote intrauterine devices (IUD) in a downscale Metro Manila community illustrates a poorly executed service delivery, and the negative consequences that this can have. One of the health centers in the community reported low acceptance rates. It explained the low turnout as something that is to be expected because women have a "natural fear of the IUD and they also know that the method has serious side effects." The program's Metro Manila headquarters could not accept the center's explanation because other centers with similar market characteristics were high performing centers.

The head office program director decided to perform a spot check. He asked his wife to disguise herself as a prospective IUD adopter and to go to the health center in question. The wife reported what happened:

> As I went inside and sat in one of the chairs by the wall, I saw a woman in the operating table closest to the door I entered. There was only one operating table separated by a movable wood divider from the doctor's office. The woman lying on the table looked agitated. I think she wanted someone to tell her what was going to happen.
>
> Then the clinic nurse came and started to prepare her for the doctor. But the nurse did not even greet her, and I saw the patient was getting more nervous. I didn't hear the nurse say any reassuring words to her. Then the doctor arrived. He too didn't say anything. He even seemed to avoid her eyes. He started by signaling with his hands that she should spread her legs wider. When she very reluctantly and very slowly did that but not fully, I saw the doctor frown and impatiently repeated his hand signal. He didn't seem to mind showing her the annoyed look on his face.
>
> Then without any warning or explanation, he just inserted the IUD applicator. I saw the woman's body drawing back in shocked

astonishment. She was on the verge of tears and was biting her lower lip from this traumatic treatment.

Consider the three elements of service delivery illustrated in the above situation. The two service personnel, or actors—the nurse and the doctor—were both unsympathetic and showed no sense of service. The service outlet, or stage, was the health center's operating room. It was crowded, there was no privacy, and other patients were allowed to wait their turn inside. The furnishings were sparse, there was no air conditioning, and the place lacked a sanitary appearance. The service performance, or staging, was noninteractive, abrupt, and traumatizing. It comes then as no surprise that this health center registered low IUD acceptance rates. The real surprise is that it had any clients at all.

Implementing Promotion and Pricing

Promotion can have three forms of advertising, adoption promotion, and selling. Health and nutrition program managers who make use of advertising agencies learn that ad agency people are very good at executing communication messages. The mass media-based nutrition education campaign in India in the late sixties demonstrated this. Instead of using conventional appeals drawing on the four-food-groups cliches, the campaign's film portion capitalized on the Indian fondness for astrology, and developed messages with the theme, "Your child's plate is his horoscope."[18]

Advertising agencies often excel in the message execution phase of mass communication campaigns. Health and nutrition programs should resort to them for this purpose. However, in developing a message to execute, advertising can be weak. This is particularly true when ad agencies draw upon focus group discussion research for uncovering the message. It has been shown that this research is more useful in generating ideas for more or better message execution than in generating ideas about a better message.[19] The results of focus group discussion research also cannot be generalized. UNESCO learned this when it used the method in designing its nutrition communication campaigns.[20]

The next form of promotion is adoption promotion. A key lesson from adoption promotion is that while the world may beat a path to the store that sells a better mousetrap, the world may decide to do this later rather than immediately. Health and nutrition programs need adoption promotion to get an adopter to act now and not to postpone a decision. Adoption promotion triggers adopters to translate their intention into action without delay. This suggests that if program managers want target adopters to adopt promptly, then they must follow up on advertising's motivating effect with adoption promotion efforts. Marketers refer to the two tasks as A&P, A for advertising and P for adoption promotion. A is not enough; it needs P to complete the job.

In its different forms, adoption promotion can be noisy and risky. It includes incentives to both adopters and service outlets such as contests, giveaways, lotteries, and special events, all of which aim to boost adoption of a product or a service. Clearly, health and nutrition program managers have to be careful in their choice and use of adoption promotion. They can also utilize another type of adoption promotion, one that "solicits the involvement and participation of target adopters, which leads to trial adoption, which, in turn can lead to committed adoption."[21] The development literature has extensively examined this adoption promotion under such names as *participative adoption* and *empowerment.*[22]

A third form of promotion is what business marketing calls *selling.* The salesman is also known as the *sales representative, salesperson, account executive, sales engineer, field rep, service rep, and marketing rep.* Social marketing calls it *personal communication.* In national development programs, on the other hand, the personal communicator is known as *extension worker, field worker, outreach worker, field motivator, community organizer, volunteer worker, service provider, social worker, field educator,* and *field counselor.* The difference in names reflects the difference in how the promotional functions are performed. Because of the increasing use in business marketing of multilevel distribution channels, selling is getting further and further removed from the ultimate consumer and more and more tied into trade intermediaries. Yet personal communication is a direct, highly interactive contact with the target adopters. This is why even when a health program, such as the Measles Vaccination Campaign in Manila, uses the term, "sales force," it suggests an aggressive campaign to win adoptions. The campaign of the Philippine Department of Health defines "sales force" as follows:

The sales force in a health communication campaign is composed of the frontliners: healthworkers who interact with mothers face-to-face. Healthworkers are a special brand of "sales force."

Their responsibility for ensuring the health of the child is far-reaching. They are "selling" a health practice, not for the "profits" they will reap from sales but out of a deep commitment to the people who must be empowered to take care of their own health."[23]

When personal communicators give their deep commitment, it is easy to understand why social marketers argue that "of the three main promotional communication tools, personal communication exercises the most powerful influence."[24]

Finally, the last P in the social marketing mix is pricing. Business marketers who have assisted in social program planning and implementation have learned that it is in the pricing area where the marketing approach needs the most modification. In social or nonprofit programs, the critical price of adoption is not monetary but nonmonetary.

Seen from the adopter's standpoint, pricing includes all the costs involved in adopting a social product. Often, the adopter's most burdensome costs are nonmonetary, such as the behavioral cost in transportation time to a health center, the waiting time, and usage or consumption time. Other nonmonetary costs can involve learning or habit-forming time, the psychological risk of product nonper-formance, the risk of stigma and embarrassment from the act of adopting, and the fear of side effects. Adopters may judge adoption unaffordable because of their perceptions of the nonmonetary, as well as monetary, costs.

Applying the Social Marketing Mix Framework

Depending on the kind of health and nutrition product involved, the social market-ing mix may be easy or difficult to put into practice. When the marketing product is a tangible one, it typically is easier than when a product is intangible.

Oral rehydration solution for diarrheal babies exemplifies a tangible health and nutrition product. Implementing the social marketing mix for this product is relatively easy; it comes very close to the business marketing setting. The target adopter segments and the adopters' needs are identifiable, using traditional busi-ness marketing tools. The intermediate adopter responses and ultimate adopter behavior are identifiable, again using traditional business marketing instruments.

Breast-feeding promotion campaigns present, on the other hand, an intangible product. Defining the product in this case raises the question of what the program wants the target adopters, i.e., the lactating mothers, to adopt. The immediate answer is that breast-feeding, as opposed to nonbreast-feeding, is the product. But how can this be a social program's product? After all, it is a practice that comes not from a program but from the actions of target adopters themselves.

Social marketing will define this product as the bundle of needs that the breast-feeding will satisfy among the target population segment of nonbreast-feed-ing mothers. However, it can be argued that mothers who are not breast-feeding are presumably satisfying their own set of needs in rejecting the practice. This means that the program's real product is the value of breast-feeding offered to the target adopters as something that will satisfy them better than the value that they now feel they gain from nonbreast-feeding. For the adopting mothers, advocates have argued that the value of breast-feeding consists of two health benefits. It improves "the nutritional and ultimately the health status of infants," and it contrib-utes "to child spacing."[25] On the other hand, mothers who have decided not to breast-feed do so because of their "need or desire to work" or return to work or because of personal beauty considerations.[26]

With intangible products such as breast-feeding or immunization practices, program implementers have to pay even greater attention to needs assessment, product analysis, and social marketing mix formulation. To be effective, imple-menting instruments may require modifying and perhaps even overhauling the marketing approach in place.

Table 6-3 summarizes the situation and highlights the need for social market-ers to

1.   identify all classes of social products involved in an intervention and locate them, analytically, along a range bounded at two ends by tangible and intangible products; and

2.   design any required modifications in the marketing mix model that are called for by the types of products, or product classes.

Organizing, Controlling, and Evaluating a Social Program

As the preceding steps are being taken, the program implementer must also organize the social marketing campaign that has to be carried out at three levels: the headquarters level, field operations level, and the support level, where cooperation from other implementing or resource-holding offices must be secured. At the headquarters level, organizing for social marketing means establishing a program management team that will bring the social marketing mix down through the organizational structure to the field and grassroots level. The idea is to maintain the integrity of the program throughout the different levels of the organization. This does not mean that the program should be inflexible to changes required by district and local variations. Maintaining program integrity does not mean insensitivity to local needs that may require modifications. It means, however, not departing from the program's fundamental objectives and its target adopter segments and beneficiaries.

At the field operations level, organizing a social marketing program means setting up the field staff that will adapt the headquarters program to the local situation. An appropriate social marketing mix can be adjusted for local requirements and yet still serve the program objectives. In reviewing traditional approaches to nutrition interventions, one study concluded that many nutrition programs do not reach "the nutritionally most vulnerable groups."[27] Neglect of, or inadequate attention to, the field operations level can explain in part this lack of coverage and the failure to reach the target beneficiaries.

Organizing at the support level can mean either of two things. First, it means coordinating activities with the other departments in the health and nutrition policy and program structure. These other departments control such important resources as operating funds, training, research, supplies, facilities, transport, and others. They are typically at the same level in the organization as the program implementing group. To get their cooperation and support, implementers must relate to them and persuade them to lend the needed support at the appropriate time, place, and in the appropriate amount.

The other meaning of organizing at the support level goes beyond coordination. It actually requires a social marketing program of its own. This is the case when support derives from influential independent organizations. For instance, a nutrition program under the Ministry of Health may need the support of other government agencies such as the Ministry of Agriculture, the Ministry of Finance, the Ministry of Public Works and Communication, or the Ministry of Education. It may also require the help of private sector organizations such as the owners, managers, and workers involved in food processing and manufacturing companies. These are complex influence groups. Conventional coordinating efforts will not be enough to get them to actively support the nutrition program as allies, or to disarm them if they happen to be opponents. To influence either of these behaviors will require a social marketing program in its own right.[28]

Together with organizing, the program implementer must attend to the task of ensuring that implementation is both timely and efficient. This is the control task. It focuses on the question of how well the program is performing relative to its objectives. The control task may require keeping activity-driven and people-driven deviations from the program's action plans within tolerable limits. This way, the program comes as close as possible to attaining the stated objectives.

It is easy to get lost in the intricacies of a control system. Techniques with engaging hardware and software abound. They meticulously track activities, inputs, and outputs. They flash early warning red lights to alert program implementers about the appearance of deviations. But this is only one side of control. It is the nonhuman side. The other side, the human side, needs as much attention from the program management. In fact, the management guru, Peter Drucker, favors a greater emphasis on the human dimension:

> [T]he ultimate control of the organization . . . lies in its people decisions. . . . Even the most powerful "instrument board," complete with computers, operations research, and simulation, is secondary to the invisible, qualitative control of any human organization, its systems of rewards and punishments, of values and taboos.[29]

In social marketing, the task of program evaluation is not the same as the control task. Control assumes that "observed performance is causally linked to the program" while evaluation precisely questions this assumption.[30] Evaluation is concerned with two additional questions: Did the nutrition program cause the observed behavior from the target adopters or was the cause some other factors? and Did the program choose the right behavior to change or sustain with the right means and social marketing mix?

The first question involves the issue of impact evaluation; the second, the issue of ethical evaluation. Both questions are a concern for the program implementer. Impact evaluation is a humbling question. There are times when it tells the implementer that the desired adopter behavior took place not really because of the program but in spite of it. Ethical evaluation raises questions about human values, in the words of one marketing veteran, "obligating marketers to work on behalf of their clients' or adopters' long-term well-being and satisfaction."[31] It keeps marketers from misusing and abusing the tools of their practice.

Successes and Failures in Program Development

Asian countries that are combatting hunger and malnutrition have used a repertoire of nutrition programs. In Thailand, for example, these embrace "a curative and primary health care program, a food supply and availability program, a nutrition education program and an income generation program."[32] In India, interventions include a food fortification program using such diverse items as bread, *atta* (a ground wheat used for making a dietary staple), salt, tea, and a tapioca product called *sago*. Other programs include a private initiative of introducing beneficial nutritious foods in the marketplace, undertaken by members of the Protein Foods Association; a school and preschool child feeding program; a mass media nutrition education program; and "a child welfare program featuring nutrition feeding of small children and pregnant and nursing women, education of the mothers, special prophylactic measures against nutritional anemia and blindness, immunization, preschool education, and health care."[33]

The success record of these programs is mixed. Some have had near complete success, others partial successes, and still others have been failures. But evaluations depend on the measure of success. One study applied a malnutrition reduction measure. It came to a disturbing conclusion: "When measured in terms of their effect on the extent of malnutrition in any country, the impact has been negligible."[34]

Analysis of the sources of failure in nutrition programs indicates that they include shortcomings such as reaching the wrong target segments ("it was not the malnourished who were accessed by these programs"), "poor referral systems," "sparse coverage and little follow-up," "inadequate maintenance," and similar other management weaknesses. These are all inadequacies of program implementation.

Conclusion

I have proposed in this paper that in order to apply the impressive gains from nutrition research, technology development, and planning and policy formulation to the ultimate target beneficiaries, namely, malnourished and unhealthy people, we have to give priority to developing program management skills and building an effective implementation process. To this end, the paper proposed and explored the implementation practice known as social marketing. A question posed at the 1988 Smithsonian food colloquium, which I referred to earlier, was: Why have we not done more "when the nutrition problem seems to be well defined, the solutions well researched, and the actions required seem to be so obviously doable?" The answer posed in this essay is that it may turn out to require as prosaic a task as doing a good job at the doable, and in the final analysis carrying out good implementation.

Notes

1. Alan Berg, *The Nutrition Factor: Its Role in National Development* (Washington, D.C.: The Brookings Institution, 1973), 210.

2. John W. Mellor, "Introduction," in *Completing the Food Chain,* ed. P. M. Hirschoff and Neil G. Kotler (Washington, D.C.: Smithsonian Institution Press, 1989), xxi.

3. Gelia T. Castillo, "Confronting the 'Nuts and Bolts' in the Food Chain," in *Completing the Food Chain,* 132.

4. "Directions for Research on Completing the Food Chain: A Discussion," in *Completing the Food Chain,* 157.

5. Berg, 8.

6. "Directions for Research on Completing the Food Chain . . ." in *Completing the Food Chain,* 161.

7. Thomas J. Peters and Robert H. Waterman, *In Search of Excellence: Lessons from America's Best-Run Companies* (New York: Harper & Row, 1982).

8. Aree Valyasevi and Pattanee Winichagoon, "Food Production and Nutrition in Southeast Asia." in *Completing the Food Chain,* 38.

9. See, for example, S. Reutlinger and M. Selowsky, *Malnutrition and Poverty* (Baltimore: Johns Hopkins Press, 1976).

10. Tina G. Sanghvi and Arun P. Sanghvi, "Factoring Nutrition in Development Planning: A Role for Management Science," in *Planning Processes in Developing Countries: Techniques and Achievements,* ed. W. D. Cook and T. E. Kuhn (Amsterdam: North-Holland Publishing, 1982), 266.

11. Edward C. Baer, "Promoting Breast-feeding: A National Responsibility," *Studies in Family Planning,* 12 (April 1981), 203.

12. Berg, 187.

13. Richard K. Manoff, *Social Marketing: New Imperatives for Public Health* (New York: Praeger, 1985), 227.

14. Manoff, 226.

15. Such an identity is made in H. A. Simon and A. Newell, "The Uses and Limitations of Models," in *Theories in Contemporary Psychology,* ed. M. H. Marx (New York: Macmillan, 1963); and in A. Kaplan, *The Conduct of Inquiry: Methodology for Behavioral Science* (New York: In-text Educational Publishers, 1964).

16. Ledivina V. Carino, "Toward More Effective Health Care for the Poor: Conclusions and Recommendations," in *Integration, Participation and Effectiveness: An Analysis of the Operations and Effects of Five Rural Health Delivery Mechanisms,* ed. L. V. Carino, et al. (Metro Manila: Philippine Institute for Development Studies, 1982), 221.

17. Eduardo L. Roberto, *Social Marketing and Its Applications: a State of the Art Review* (Washington, D.C.: The World Bank, 1988), 29.

18. Berg, 187.

19. See Chapter 7 in Eduardo L. Roberto, *Applied Marketing Research* (Metro Manila: Ateneo University Press, 1987).

20. Ronal C. Israel, *Operational Guidelines for Social Marketing Projects in Public Health and Nutrition* (Paris: UNESCO, 1987).

21. Philip Kotler and Eduardo L. Roberto, *Social Marketing: Strategies for Changing Public Behavior* (New York: The Free Press, 1989).

22. See, for example, Carlos A. Fernandes, *Lessons in Self-Reliance and Empowerment* (Metro Manila: Foundation for the Advancement of Filipino Women, 1985); and Frances Korten, "Community Participation: a Management Perspective on Obstacles and Options," in *Bureaucracy and the Poor: Closing the Gap,* ed. D. C. Korten and F. B. Alfonso (Singapore: McGraw-Hill International Book Co., 1981).

23. Cecilia Cabanero-Verzosa, *Managing a Communication Program on Immunization* (Washington, D.C.: Academy for Educational Development, 1989), 33.

24. Kotler and Roberto, 221–22.

25. Penny Van Estrik and Ted Greiner, "Breast-feeding and Women's Work: Constraints and Opportunities," *Studies in Family Planning* 12 (April 1981), 184–97.

26. Nestle Company, *Infant Nutrition in Developing Countries: A Nestle Viewpoint* (White Plains, New York: Nestle Co., no date), 17.

27. Sanghvi and Sanghvi, 258.

28. For a discussion of the elements in the social marketing to influence groups, see Chapter 15 of Kotler and Roberto.

29. Peter F. Drucker, *Management: Tasks, Responsibilities, Practices* (New York: Harper & Row, 1974), 504.

30. Eduardo L. Roberto, *Strategic Decision Making in a Social Program* (Lexington, Mass.: Lexington Books, 1975), 112.

31. Philip Kotler, "Humanistic Marketing: Beyond the Marketing Concept," in *Philosophical and Radical Thoughts in Marketing,* ed. A. F. Firat, N. Dholakia, and R. P. Bagozzi (Lexington, Mass.: Lexington Books, 1987), 271–88.

32. Valyasevi and Winichagoon, 38.

33. Berg, 188.

34. Sanghvi and Sanghvi, 258.

CHAPTER 7

Frontiers of Nutrition and Food Security in Asia, Africa, and Latin America: A Colloquium Summation

Barbara A. Underwood
Assistant Director for International Program Activities,
National Eye Institute
National Institutes of Health
Bethesda, Maryland

Malnutrition still prevails in Asia, Africa, and Latin America at unconscionable levels and takes its toll in human life, misery and, in my view, in human dignity. As Peter Greaves reminded us, we recently experienced in New York an unprecedented United Nations Summit for Children in which more than seventy world leaders and over eighty country representatives met for two days and focused on the global campaign to erase, and I quote a newspaper, "the hunger, illness, and continuous poverty faced by tens of millions of the world's children." And I want to add to that—"and their families." But, will this turn out to be yet another two-day road show? Let's hope not. This colloquium perhaps represents a modest extension of that summit effort.

We have been privileged to hear the ideas and experiences of scientists, medical doctors, and policy specialists who have struggled with the problems of malnutrition and disease in their own countries and regions, and who have worked with national programs and international agencies that seek to improve the situation. They have reported to us some successful experiences and some not so successful. Yet, lessons can be drawn from all of these to guide us in our future efforts.

I was very encouraged that such efforts are, in fact, under way. Dr. Rahmathullah related to us how raising the level of nutrition for one nutrient, vitamin A, among deficient, chronically undernourished preschool children can have a very dramatic effect on their chances of surviving even common infections such as diarrhea and measles. She also pointed out, however, that it will take more than supplying a single nutrient to substantially improve child health. A broader attack

---

Editor's note: Dr. Underwood's summation was taped, transcribed, and edited for publication.

is needed on the surrounding conditions of poverty and deprivation to prevent and to reduce the frequency at which infectious illnesses occur. Her presentation emphasized that in India and elsewhere where the health infrastructure often is lacking in reach and coverage for the purposes of effective nutrition interventions, it becomes necessary to integrate strategies for ensuring an adequate intake of vitamin A into existing community-based programs. Exemplifying this need are programs that serve meals to children or have contact with the families of children, particularly those in the first three years of life.

An adequate diet containing vitamin A is the preferred route of intervention, Dr. Rahmathullah observed. To attain this on a sustainable basis in India involves the assurance of household food security, and this can only be achieved by involving the agricultural sector in human development issues. Agriculturalists need to be more aware of what is doable at the household level with their help in making vitamin A-rich foods available through home gardening and at affordable prices in local rural markets, as well as in urban centers.

The People's Republic of China, the largest country in Asia both in area and in population, is confronted with the serious public health problem of iron deficiency, which Dr. Liu related to us. This problem afflicts many other countries both in the developing world and in the developed world. Dr. Liu not only described the magnitude of the problem and its causes among Chinese children and women, but also outlined a wide range of strategies being undertaken in China to prevent or combat this fully remediable human health disorder. She stressed that nutrition education is an important strategy for the eradication of iron deficiency, and by this statement she meant formal training and education of health professionals as well as instruction at the household level so that the appropriate information could become an integral part of food, nutrition, and community health programs.

Problems of child malnutrition continue to plague and even increase in magnitude in parts of Africa. Miss Maribe attributed this to the continuing unresolved problems inherent in the African food system. She noted that the concept of food security is still not understood, even among the graduates of health, food, and nutrition programs who are educated in the countries within the region, thus indicating the need in Africa for both human and institutional capacity building.

The East, Central and Southern Africa Food and Nutrition Cooperative Group that she is working with is a very promising organization for addressing the problems of malnutrition and hunger. The group is providing interagency collaboration with a regional focus to help develop complementary project linkages that strengthen country and regional-level food systems. She emphasized a point also made by Dr. Rahmathullah that improvements as a result of health-specific interventions will be limited unless activities outside the health sector, particularly those involving agriculture, also are brought into the mainstream and are targeted to the underserved areas and households. Miss Maribe pointed out that improvement in nutritional status must become an explicit objective of development policies at the regional, national, and local levels.

Dr. Roberto reminded us that the knowledge base, the techniques, and the technology for solving nutrition problems have existed for at least a decade. Yet, only two years ago at a previous Smithsonian colloquium Gelia Castillo, the noted Philippine sociologist, asked, why haven't we done more for health and nutrition, since the actions required seem so obviously doable? Dr. Roberto contends that the key is to actually start doing the doable well, to start implementing well interventions of whatever kind, and that is where the management practice he represents, known as social marketing, can make a contribution.

Dr. Roberto believes that implementation is often taken for granted and that our best talents and skills are frequently not applied to the implementation process as they are to research, technology, development and planning, and policy formulation. Yet, good implementation requires a systematic approach to doing the doable well. And this calls for the appropriate mix of social marketing techniques. He emphasized that it is this total mix of techniques that must be created and applied in shaping behaviors and responses for improved health and nutrition among targeted segments of the population.

Dr. Monckeberg described the example of a country that has made remarkable progress in doing the doable. Notable achievements have been made in Chile in improving health, nutrition, and the quality of life over the past couple of decades. This has occurred without much progress in the nation's economic development. He attributed much of the success to a political decision to protect and develop the human resources of Chile, which he considers the most important factor of development. (I pause here to note that not only did Dr. Monckeberg voice this view but most of the other speakers also emphasized the importance of human resource development.) The extremely poor in any country, Dr. Monckeberg contends, have no voice, no expectations, no capacity to organize or ability to exert political pressure to better their own lives. They require a basic national health infrastructure if their health needs are to be met. Chile started such a scheme in the early 1950s, and I had not realized that Dr. Abraham Horwitz was closely involved in those early days in its development. Dr. Horwitz is very much to be commended for helping to initiate this remarkable example of a successful, sustainable, national public health program.

Dr. Monckeberg described to us how the health service in Chile has extended its scope and coverage in recent years under the guidance, and with the cooperation, of private and university groups. He noted that the program extends beyond simply distributing milk and other nutrition supplements; it also addresses other basic issues that influence health and nutrition, such as child care, education, female literacy, household and environmental sanitation, and a more equitable agricultural policy. Yet, what has been achieved in Chile through a national health service delivery system has not been successfully achieved in some of the other countries, as Dr. Rahmathullah pointed out.

Recently, James Grant, executive director of UNICEF, made the following statement, and I quote: "Each of the great social achievements of recent decades has come about not because of government proclamations but because people organized, made demands, and made it good politics for governments to respond." I've tried to extract from today's discussion some of the ideas put forward that might facilitate, as Dr. Rahmathullah put it, "a people's movement toward the improvement of their own lot" and to which governments would feel it would be good politics to respond. What are the factors that, even under the prevailing conditions of poverty, have nudged forward the movement toward food security and have helped to reduce undernutrition? Let me suggest the following:

1. Awareness   This perhaps is the most critical component needed to obtain acceptance to start a program and to sustain it. It is essential to create this awareness at all levels—the government leaders at the national level, those at the local level, and down to the members of each household. Each level must recognize that there is a problem and that there are doable solutions available.

2. Choice   People, regardless of their socioeconomic status, like to choose from alternatives in matters that affect their lives. Usually there is a range of possible solutions, some doable through national initiatives, others at the community level, and yet others at the household level. Too often the choice is made by those external to the situation and without local consultation. We, those of us at higher decision-making levels, are convinced that we have to do the doable for them, rather than allowing them to become the doers!

3. Empowerment   Some may have a better word for this, but the concept involves the ability to control conditions locally that affect the well-being of the nation, community, or household, in other words, self-reliance. I think that this message came through clearly in the presentations, the need nationally and locally to minimize external dependence. Empowerment at all levels within a country is needed, but added empowerment should be the particular goal at the community and household levels. It is of paramount importance for these people to realize how the doable is done by the people themselves, and not by someone else for them or to them. For this empowerment to occur, local people must have knowledge as to what is doable within their context, and how (usually they do know but are not heard!), and they must have the needed resources made available to do the doable where feasible for themselves.

4. Public demand   Public awareness that benefits can accrue creates a demand and, in turn, can lead to political pressure for action. To draw again on a quote from Jim Grant: "It is the political will of the people that makes and sustains the political will of government." Those who are too often the recipients of our well-meaning nutrition and health interventions and programs, as Dr. Roberto observed, have got to become the consumers. They must view these programs we are trying to impose upon them as being in their best interests, thus creating a demand for services. Dr. Monckeberg argued that in order for this to happen, nutrition and health must be made a political issue. The World Health Organization estimates that fifteen million children die annually around the world and that currently three to four

million are saved by various health interventions. The global objective is to double that number.

As we have heard today, health and nutrition interventions for maximum impact must address the underlying issues of poverty and underdevelopment, among which one of the most prominent is household food security—a complex issue that goes beyond that usually addressed within the health system. Therefore, to address this complex issue in sustainable, effective ways requires a multidisciplinary, multisectoral involvement at the regional, national, and local levels. Furthermore, as others have said, it requires putting a human face on development policy planning and programs, regardless of the sector or discipline.

In this colloquium it has been repeatedly emphasized that food, nutrition, and health programs should not exist as vertical programs within the health ministry, nor should agricultural programs be solely production-oriented, thereby ignoring consumption issues, household food security, and community nutritional needs. Indeed, as Miss Maribe has suggested, health, nutrition, and food security are inextricably interrelated and must become explicit objectives of development policies, particularly agricultural development policy.

I want to conclude by thanking our host for inviting me to participate in the colloquium today. It has been a very good learning experience for me and, I hope, for all of us.

CHAPTER 8

The Role of the Potato in the Conquest of Hunger

John S. Niederhauser
1990 World Food Prize Laureate
Tucson, Arizona

I am deeply honored to be the 1990 World Food Prize laureate. It is with a genuine feeling of both pride and humility that I accept this award. My feeling of pride is based on the knowledge that this award recognizes the contributions made not only by me but also by my colleagues and friends all over the world, working together for so many years. And I am proud to accept this award in their name as well. I feel humble because I am joining the company of distinguished laureates who have been honored in the previous three years: M. S. Swaminathan, Robert Chandler, Jr., and Verghese Kurien.

At this time I am sure that all of us will join me in expressing our appreciation to Norman Borlaug, whose inspiration led to the creation of the World Food Prize. We are also grateful to the Council of Advisors and the sponsors who have established and guided the Prize.

I wish to call your attention at this time to one very special person who has been a constant source of support and encouragement during my career. Not only has she travelled with me all over the world and shared the satisfaction of cooperating with our colleagues in so many countries, but she has created the home and family that have made my life so wonderful. Those of you who know her are aware of how vital she has been to whatever might have been accomplished. I would like to introduce this person who shares with me the honor of the 1990 World Food Prize, my wife Ann Niederhauser.

Editor's note: The following are the remarks of John S. Niederhauser on the occasion of accepting the award of the World Food Prize, which took place at the Smithsonian Institution's Baird Auditorium, October 17, 1990. The remarks have been edited and expanded, with graphs and tables, for inclusion in this volume. A version of this essay appeared in *Arizona Land and People* [College of Agriculture, University of Arizona] 40, 4 (Winter 1990).

In 1947 I began my career in international agricultural cooperation and development as the plant pathologist on a small team of scientists sent by the Rockefeller Foundation to Mexico. Our purpose was to work with the Mexican government in a national program to increase production of basic food crops in that country. This innovative program was one of the first ventures in international agricultural assistance. Under the leadership of Dr. George Harrar, this Mexican agricultural program was a pioneering model in the establishment of other agricultural assistance programs throughout the world under the sponsorship of many agencies. The national wheat, maize, and potato programs developed in Mexico soon acquired regional and then international dimensions. A similar strategy was subsequently established to increase rice production in Asia, and these programs together led to the creation in the 1960s of the first International Agricultural Research Center.

Increasing Potato Production in the Developing World

The Mexican National Potato Program was launched in 1948. This production-oriented effort from the beginning emphasized collaboration with farmers, who applied both established and new technologies to improve potato yields. This highly successful national program led to a sixfold increase in potato production in Mexico from 1950 to 1980 (Figure 8-1). The value of the increase in annual potato production was over ten times the total thirty-year budget of the national potato program from 1950 to 1980.

The Mexican National Potato Program also played a vital role as an operating and training base in the development of national potato programs throughout the Third World. Using the same field-oriented approach that was proving so successful in Mexico, we were able to work with farmers, scientists, and decision-makers to improve potato production in many countries.

Over 180 scientists from developing countries participated in potato production and training activities based in the Mexican National Potato Program. The leaders of potato programs in twenty-seven countries had the opportunity to visit Mexico and work in the field with their Mexican colleagues for periods of six to twelve months, including at least one complete growing season of the potato crop. Successful working relationships multiplied among these potato programs all over the world.

By 1956 an Inter-American Potato Program had been established on the basis of the collaboration of national potato programs throughout Latin America. The International Potato Program, based in Mexico and supported by international funding, was formed in 1961 to stimulate increases in national potato production in many Third World countries.

Figure 8-1

Increases in Potato Planting Area, Production, and Yield in Mexico, 1952–1980

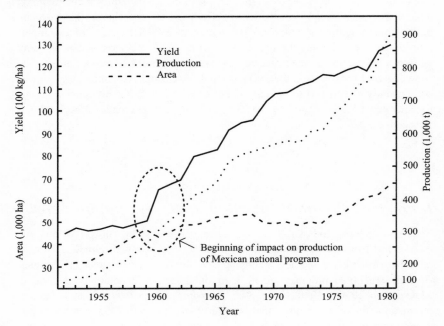

Source: Direccion General de Economia Agricola, Secretaria de Agricultura y Ganaderia, Annual Reports, 1953–1981; FAO Production Yearbook, 1955–1985.

National potato program development in these countries followed a similar pattern:

1.   Identification of program priorities and production restraints;

2.   Emphasis on production-oriented research and on intense cooperative effort to demonstrate improved production technology directly in farmers' fields;

3.   Collaboration among national institutions, personnel, and between production sectors and decision makers, in accordance with their priorities, so as to promote a more efficient utilization of scarce resources and to avoid duplication of effort;

4.   Recognition that increases in productivity depend upon close cooperation among farmers, scientists, and technologists.

Modest budgets and limited personnel obliged the International Potato Program to work with and through the national potato programs. In retrospect, the ostensible constraints, both in resources and in facilities, made necessary a cooperative production strategy that was itself directly responsible for the dramatic increases in the productivity and continuity of these national potato programs in developing countries throughout the world.

The need for establishing the International Potato Program as a strong institution in the world became increasingly apparent, and in 1971 the International Potato Center (Centro Internacional de la Papa, CIP) was created in Lima, Peru. The existing international program and its regional components formed the operating base of this new center. During its two decades of growth, CIP has become a prominent research and development center as a result of having a set of characteristics that was inherited from the International Potato Program that preceded it:

1. A modest headquarters;
2. Efficient use of contract research, making use of the strength and excellence of research institutions in the United States and Europe, as needed and appropriate;
3. Regionalization of programs, with emphasis on the building of strength and continuity in national programs;
4. Maintenance of a large-scale germplasm bank in several locations, both to be utilized in current potato breeding programs and to be conserved for future needs.

The value of this strategy in international cooperation and development is widely recognized today. In 1986, at the twentieth anniversary celebration of the International Corn and Wheat Improvement Center in Mexico, Dr. S. Husain, chairman of the Consultative Group on International Agricultural Research (CGIAR), paid tribute to

> the pioneering relationship between the farsighted agricultural research
> program of Mexico and a small group of Rockefeller Foundation scien-
> tists. The entire CGIAR system owes its existence to the approach used in
> the Mexico-Rockefeller Program—that of scientists from different
> countries working together to solve major agricultural problems.[1]

During the past thirty years, total potato production in the developing countries of the world has tripled. This is due to a 50 percent increase in the acreage planted, and, even more important, to a 100 percent increase in productivity, or yield per hectare. In 1950, less than 4 percent of world potato production was located in the developing countries. Today, it is nearly 15 percent (Table 8-1). It is to be noted that the rate of increase in potato production in the Third World is greater than for any other major food crop.

The best measure of the impact of successful national potato programs in a sampling of five countries, as shown in Table 8-2, is not just the significant increase in production that has occurred in the last few decades. There also has been a 70 to 100 percent increase in per capita potato consumption annually in these five countries during the past thirty years. Even though potato consumption in these countries still is much lower than in Europe or the United States, the potato is becoming a much more important food crop in these countries, where it is now recognized to be a valuable source of nutrients, and no longer is considered to be merely an expensive vegetable.

Table 8-1

World Potato Area, Production, and Yield, 1948–52, 1984

	Area (1,000,000 ha)		Production (1,000,000 t)		Yield (t/ha)	
	1948–52	**1984**	**1948–52**	**1984**	**1948–52**	**1984**
World	22.6	20.3	247.4	312.2	11.0	15.4
Industrialized	21.1	17.0	238.3	272.4	11.3	16.0
Nonindustrialized	1.5	3.3	9.1	39.8	6.2	12.1

Sources: FAO Production Yearbooks (Rome: Food and Agriculture Organization, 1960, 1970, 1975, 1983, 1985, and 1988); and D. Horton and Hugo Fano, *Potato Atlas* (Lima, Peru: International Potato Center, 1985).

This success story is the result of an international cooperative effort involving potato farmers, scientists, and decision-makers in national programs all over the world. All of them can take justifiable pride in the growing contribution that the potato is making to the world food supply.

PRECODEPA: A New Strategy in Regional Cooperation for the Transfer of Technology

During the 1970s, the national resources available for agricultural research and development were very limited in many developing countries. Often it has not been possible to finance a complete national crop production program with all of the needed technical personnel and components. To alleviate the problems caused by this lack of funds and personnel, the Programa Regional Cooperativo de Papa (PRECODEPA) project was launched in 1978 at a regional meeting attended by representatives from Guatemala, Mexico, Honduras, Costa Rica, Panama, Dominican Republic, and from the International Potato Center.[2] Today there are ten countries participating in PRECODEPA, with CIP as the eleventh member.

At the organizational meeting in Guatemala, each country listed the factors that limited potato production and productivity in that country. Most of these limiting factors were common to several of the countries: the availability of good seed; late blight resistance; low-cost rustic storage, and similar problems. The regional program, PRECODEPA, was organized to help solve through regional cooperation the problems associated with each of the limiting factors. Leadership for the projects was assigned to one of the collaborating national programs, which, with international financial support, developed the personnel, research, and materials for the solution of that particular production problem. The research technology and training opportunities derived from these PRECODEPA projects were shared with each interested country. Among the direct benefits to the participating national programs have been the increases in potato production and productivity, greater continuity in national program activities and personnel, and more efficient utilization of scarce resources.

Table 8-2

Annual Increases in Potato Production in Selected Countries, 1948–1982

Country	1948–52			1978–82		
	Area (1,000 ha)	**Production** (1,000 t)	**Yield** (t/ha)	**Area** (1,000 ha)	**Production** (1,000 t)	**Yield** (t/ha)
Bangladesh	50	250	5.0	109	1,150	10.6
Colombia	55	506	9.2	168	2,190	13.0
India	277	1,547	6.8	806	12,250	15.2
Mexico	30	134	4.5	69	1,094	15.8
Turkey	79	605	7.7	190	3,200	16.8

Sources: FAO Production Yearbook, (Rome: Food and Agriculture Organization, 1960, 1983); *and* D. Horton and Hugo Fano, *Potato Atlas* (Lima, Peru: International Potato Center, 1985).

PRECODEPA is governed by a committee composed of one representative from each participating country and from CIP. All regional activities are financed by international funds, which to date have been supplied by the Swiss government. Activities that are strictly national in scope continue to be financed by national funds.

PRECODEPA has been recognized as a very cost-efficient strategy for improving agricultural production and productivity in countries with limited resources, and has served as a model for similar cooperative programs in other regions of the world. Many of us feel that PRECODEPA could become the most important new development in the transfer of agricultural technology since the creation of the International Agricultural Research Centers.

PICTIPAPA: A New Strategy to Control Potato Late Blight

The potato production breakthroughs during the past few decades have significantly boosted yield, yet in recent years potato production has leveled off in many developing countries. There is an explanation for this loss of momentum.

If the potato is to be grown more widely in the world, and its potential as a food crop in developing countries to be fully realized, resistance to the late blight disease is essential. Wherever potatoes are grown under rainfall, the susceptible varieties must be protected by fungicides, which are expensive and often unavailable in Third World countries. In some regions, farmers try to avoid late blight by growing potatoes under irrigation during the dry season. But irrigated land is becoming increasingly expensive and scarce. Developing a resistance to late blight is the obvious solution if the potato is to become an important staple food in these countries.

For more than a century since the late blight disease devastated the potato crop in Ireland and caused the tragic famine there, the search for a durable resistance to this plague has proved to be frustrating and largely unsuccessful. In potato breeding programs all over the world, the story was the same: soon after supposedly resistant potato cultivars were developed and released, they fell susceptible to new races of the causal fungus pathogen.

Early in the development of the Mexican National Potato Program, it was discovered that Mexico had some unique advantages for the study of this most important disease of potatoes.[3] First, Mexico was the native home of the wild potato species that had been used in worldwide potato breeding programs as the source of late blight resistance. Second, Mexico was discovered to be the place of origin of the fungus pathogen, *Phytophthora infestans.*

The Mexican potato breeding program soon became a world center for the study of potato late blight, and for the development of potato cultivars with a durable horizontal resistance to this disease. The historic contributions of Mexican-based research on potato late blight have greatly improved the chances for success in the worldwide search for the control of this disease through the use of resistant potato cultivars.

Today, the Mexican National Potato Program has about twenty-five potato varieties with high levels of a durable resistance to late blight. Several of these varieties have been grown successfully for more than twenty years by subsistence farmers in the mountains of central Mexico, and grown without the application of expensive fungicides. Other blight-resistant Mexican potato varieties have been grown for a number of years in other Third World countries, such as the Philippines, Nepal, and Guatemala. The Mexican cultivars have made a substantial contribution to the food supply in these countries.

There still remains an enormous, unexploited potential for increased food production in many countries of the developing world that can be met through the expanded cultivation of blight-resistant potato cultivars. These new Mexican potato varieties have the potential to become the most promising plant materials for expanding world food production since the introduction in the Green Revolution a few decades ago of the short-strawed, rust-resistant wheats and the "miracle rice" varieties. The Mexican blight-resistant potato varieties could, indeed, ignite a new

Green Revolution, in fact, an even greener revolution than the preceding, since it would be accomplished with fewer chemicals, rather than more.

To help realize more of this potential for world food production, a new international cooperative program was launched in August 1990 by the Mexican Ministry of Agriculture, in collaboration with scientists from Poland, the Netherlands, Canada, the United States, Mexico, and CIP. This new cooperative strategy, known as Programa Internacional Cooperativo del Tizon Tardio de la Papa (PICTIPAPA), will promote projects of mutual benefit to the participants, and is open to interested institutions and scientists anywhere in the world.

PICTIPAPA will provide new channels for funding and collaboration in the development of a worldwide control of the late blight disease that has plagued potato production for so many years. Among these projects is an international field trial for the testing, distribution, and multiplication of blight-resistant potato varieties throughout the world, thus making them available to subsistence farmers in every interested country.

PICTIPAPA also is of vital interest to potato scientists and farmers in the industrialized countries of the world, where 85 percent of the world potato crop is produced. These countries are concerned because a new strain of the late blight pathogen has escaped from Mexico during the past decade, and has become established throughout the world. This new strain makes it critically important for potato producers in all countries to have new varieties with higher levels of durable resistance to late blight. This can be accomplished most quickly and reliably in collaboration with the Mexican-based PICTIPAPA. Much remains to be done, but there is more hope and optimism than ever before that this 150-year-old menace to world potato production can finally be controlled.

The Conquest of Hunger

The previous three World Food Prize laureates have reported on the dramatic breakthroughs made in wheat, rice, and milk production during the past few decades. These remarkable programs have led to major increases in food availability in the world. No longer are we facing frequent famines due primarily to a lack of food. Today we are assured that there is sufficient food produced to feed the world's population. But then, paradoxically, we also are told that there are more hungry people in the world today than thirty years ago!

It is obvious that merely producing enough food is not an automatic solution to hunger. There are other problems causing food shortages and hunger. Yet the fact that the world has an adequate supply of food does give us the opportunity to confront these other problems. Hopefully, we shall have the wisdom and the time to solve them. Certainly, there is no time for complacency. Let me briefly identify two of these problems that must be solved in order to eradicate hunger and malnutrition.

Population Stabilization

Any short-term benefits from increases in food production will ultimately be nullified unless we can bring about world population stabilization. Prime Minister Jawaharlal Nehru, when discussing several of India's critical problems some thirty years ago, included the need for population stabilization among them. Then he added: "Population stabilization will not solve any of our pressing problems; but none of these problems can be solved without it."

In 1970, Dr. Norman Borlaug was awarded the Nobel Peace Prize for his leadership role in the Green Revolution. In his acceptance speech, he responded to some overly optimistic comments that the problem of world hunger had been solved: "If fully implemented, the Green Revolution can provide sufficient food for sustenance during the next three decades; but the frightening power of human reproduction must also be curbed. Otherwise the success of the Green Revolution will be ephemeral only."[4]

We are now entering the third decade following this prophetic statement. Today, the world population is more than five billion. By the end of this century it will exceed six billion. There are predictions it will stabilize by the year 2100, at a population of twelve billion. It is important to realize that approximately 90 percent of this population of twelve billion in the year 2100 will reside in what are now called the developing countries of the world.

Do our leaders have the information, planning skills, and determination to implement and enforce the policies and measures needed to achieve population stabilization by the year 2100? During this next century, can we feed this growing population while maintaining sustainable agriculture that preserves the quality of our environment? Will population stabilization be at a level consistent with the available food supply? Reliable answers to these questions are urgently needed, because the world cannot wait.

Food Distribution

According to estimates of the Food and Agriculture Organization (FAO), approximately 20 percent of the population in developing countries is suffering from hunger. Yet FAO also affirms that there is plenty of food produced in the world to feed everyone, and with some to spare. What is wrong?

The problem is one of distribution. It is beyond the scope of this brief talk to analyze the complex reasons why there can be hunger in a country that can produce an adequate food supply for its people. The causes may be economic, political, or social. But whatever the factors are that contribute to hunger, chief among them are a lack of purchasing power and poverty. This is true for any country in the world, whether developed or developing.

This is the great challenge to the world today as we proceed toward conquering hunger. How can we attain world population stabilization during the next century and, at the same time, produce adequate food for the world's population? How can we assure that food is available and accessible to all people? To reach these goals will require a coordinated and cooperative international campaign implemented by dedicated leaders and their constituencies, who understand the close relationship of population stabilization and effective food distribution in the successful conquest of hunger.

Are we equal to this challenge? As an agriculturist who has worked in farmers' fields and in research laboratories in many countries for over fifty years, I do believe that we have the soils, water resources, climates, and the technology to feed the world as it approaches population stabilization in the next century. However, it still is an open question whether we have the understanding, the dedication, and the sense of urgency needed to cooperate in a global program to feed more people and to feed people more.

We are living now in one of the most exciting and critical periods in human history. As we approach the biological limits that this planet can support, we are made even more aware that we are living in one common world. As citizens of one world, we must all work together to build a world without hunger, and at the same time conserve our environment and our energy resources.

I ask again. Are we equal to this challenge?

Notes

1.   S. Husain, "Remarks," *Centro Internacional de Mejoramiento de Maiz y Trigo's Twentieth Anniversary: A Commemoration [September 22, 1986]* (Mexico City: CIMMYT, 1986).

2.   John S. Niederhauser and M. Villarreal, "PRECODEPA, A Successful Model for a New Concept in Regional Cooperation for International Agricultural Development," *American Potato Journal* 63(1986):237–240.

3.   John S. Niederhauser, "*Phytophthora infestans:* The Mexican Connection," Plenary Session paper presented September 1989 at International Phytophthora Symposium, Dublin, Ireland.

4.   Norman E. Borlaug, "The Green Revolution, Peace, and Humanity," Speech delivered at the 1970 presentation of the Nobel Peace Prize at Oslo University.

CHAPTER 9

Excerpts from the Discussions
at the Morning and Afternoon Sessions

Morning Discussion

Barbara Underwood: We are fortunate to have two people, Dr. Greaves and Dr. McGuire, who come to us from international agencies, to comment upon and discuss the papers. Dr. Peter Greaves is with the United Nations Children's Fund (UNICEF). He is stationed now in New York but has held several posts in different parts of the world. His major responsibilities are in the micronutrient area. Dr. Greaves.

Peter Greaves: Thank you very much. This morning we have been hearing about action, studies leading to action. As they say in the subcontinent, "research, then action." That approach is very attractive to an agency such as UNICEF. It is also very appropriate in view of the remarkable event that took place two weeks ago in New York.

Seventy heads of state and representatives of countries met at the World Summit For Children and signed a document, "The Declaration and the Plan of Action." And let me remind you that the plan says, "We commit ourselves to the following ten-point program to protect the rights of children and to improve their lives." One of those ten points says, "We will work for optimal growth and

Editor's Note: The colloquium speakers presented their papers in a morning and an afternoon session. Following the papers in each of the sessions, a panel discussion was convened to examine further the issues and ideas presented in the papers and to encourage an exchange of ideas among the speakers, the discussants, and the audience. The following excerpts from the transcripts of the two panel discussions have been edited to improve their clarity and to highlight the context of the discussions. Barbara A. Underwood served as the chairperson of the morning panel, and Norge W. Jerome, of the afternoon panel.

development in childhood through measures to eradicate hunger, malnutrition, and famine, and thus to relieve millions of children of tragic suffering in a world that has the means to feed all its citizens." In the more detailed plan of action these leaders agreed to the following goals: "With the right policies, appropriate institutional arrangements and political priorities, the world is now in a position to feed all the world's children and to overcome the worst forms of malnutrition, i.e., drastically to reduce diseases that contribute to malnutrition, to cut in half protein-energy malnutrition, virtually to eliminate vitamin A deficiency and iodine-deficiency disorders, and to reduce nutritional anemia significantly."

No longer can we shrug off the ineffectiveness of programs by saying, "there's no political will." Perhaps that was always a bit simplistic. The summit demonstrates a political will in a totally new dimension. The challenge now, of course, is to translate that into action, which is back to the theme as I perceived it in this morning's papers.

Dr. Rahmathullah's important and eloquent paper described work which led her to make very precise, specific, relevant recommendations of what could be done in India, and many of these are appropriate elsewhere. It is not meant as criticism to point out that the recent recognition of the important consequences of subclinical vitamin A deficiency is more aptly described as a rediscovery. After all, vitamin A was referred to seventy or eighty years ago by those who first discovered it as the anti-infection vitamin. Yet this historical perspective does not detract in any way from the importance of demonstrating quantitatively today the consequences of such a deficiency.

Specific suggestions for action have emerged from the work in India. The first is recognition of the importance of increasing consumption of vitamin A-containing foods in the early years of life or else providing vitamin A supplementation at safe levels. This can be done effectively through community-based programs and community- and household-level actions to control infection, improve sanitation, and strengthen healthful child care practices. Attention to these three elements—household food security, health security, and child care—I deem to be profoundly important, and I will return to this a little later.

There is much emphasis given to safe dosage. But I would suggest, however, that in many places this might involve a major logistical problem. Do you see any room for higher doses? It seems to me that this still has a role to play in certain places. I suspect you may think so because you made the wise remark that there is no single way to deal with this problem. As an example, UNICEF has just provided at the request of the government of India a new capsule for vitamin A. The normal capsule is two hundred thousand units. What they have asked for is a capsule for one hundred thousand units, probably to be administered at the time when children are given vaccinations and immunizations.

But I find it personally difficult to accept the notion that the provision of supplements outside the health system always requires the so-called safe dosage level. Are health workers the only responsible people? Couldn't teachers be trained to do this? Some other kind of extension worker, in some cases a party worker, may also be appropriate. I think the health care profession has to learn to work with others if primary health care is to be successful. The Rahmathullah paper makes a very important reference to the importance of regular and systematic contact with local workers. This contact, an essential element of this kind of approach, seldom seems to be an operational objective in programming though it is a condition for successful growth monitoring and for nutrition education that aims to influence behavior.

This probably means that there has to be a facility for home visiting. The Anganwadi workers, women who work in preschool education and who are increasingly involved in providing child health care, would be able to undertake home visiting, according to the original framers of the Integrated Child Development Service (ICDS) scheme in India. It was interpreted that help might be forthcoming from the village community to take on some of the chores. That has not happened very much but it seems to me to be something very well worth pursuing. In fact, if we are serious about reaching the presently unreached groups in the population, it seems to me one has to grapple with this problem of home visiting. The study showed that the protection effect of the vitamin A supplement was most pronounced in children under one year of age. So I would deduce from that that perhaps we should start providing vitamin A in one form or another as early as possible.

Let me illustrate this with a form of technology that we are working on along with the World Health Organization (WHO)—the development of this little dispenser I have in my hand, a little bottle which contains a concentration of vitamin A. You can turn it upside down to use it so you don't have the problem of a residue remaining at the bottom of the bottle. This device can inject half a milligram into the mouth of a child. This is being tried out in various countries at the present time, and the results will be available in the near future. I think this is going to facilitate the delivery of vitamin A in the immunization context.

I liked very much the emphasis on horticulture and what might be done in that way. But I am reminded that as with everything, I suppose, people have been saying this for a long time. Several applied nutrition programs around the world have argued for this sort of thing. In India that is certainly the case. I remember when I was in India seeing a very ingenious play that communicated the virtues of the drumstick tree. This tree is all over the place, full of carotene, but not often cultivated. The question arises, why wasn't more done about cultivating such plants? That is what we have got to know and maybe you put your finger on part of it. Perhaps there wasn't sufficient support from the extension service and from the Ministry of Agriculture. Perhaps the value of techniques such as social marketing, which can bring about behavior change, was not understood in those days. Agricultural production, in other words, is not enough in itself but it is vital. The longest journey, it is said, begins with the first step. It's important to develop horticultural practices, but in countries where this is a problem, it is necessary to encourage more effective micronutrient supplementation.

The paper puts much emphasis on communication, on relevant health and nutrition education, the use of the mass media, the special effectiveness of one-on-one communication, the contact opportunity, and on the building of a people's movement. I like the phrase, "operated by people for their own development." Brave words. But how is this done? The key may be, and the third paper talks a bit about this, the local generation of information along with training so that people can assess a situation, analyze its causes, and take appropriate action. This process has come to be known, at UNICEF, as the Triple A cycle—assessment, analysis, action. The term was coined in the Iringa nutrition program in Tanzania.

Dr. Liu made some very interesting, practical suggestions for action, arising out of the extremely important work in the People's Republic of China. I would like to know more about the dietary part of it. How practical is it, in the culture of China and elsewhere, to introduce changes so that people in fact actually do consume more animal food? It is a critically important point from your studies. Or consider this: everybody drinks tea with meals, it's part of the ritual. But we know it is bad from a nutritional point of view. Is there evidence that there has been some success in dissuading people from continuing with their tea habit? That would be very useful to know.

Dr. Liu talked about the use of salt as a vehicle for iron in China and elsewhere—and I agree. But the fact of the matter is that in much of China iodine is being added to salt, and in India it is mandatory that all salt by 1992 should have iodine added to it. For this reason, the work on fortification with iron, unless it is done in the context of double fortification with both iron and iodine—which happens to present technical problems—does not really address a practical and real situation. If there is time for further comment on that, I think it would be very useful.

Miss Maribe referred to control of iodine deficiency. I'm very glad you did because it gives me an opportunity to make reference to what I think is one of the most doable activities—namely, the control of a micronutrient that can be controlled most readily and that is often overlooked. I would like to have seen this colloquium solicit a paper specifically on iodine-deficiency control. It often gets passed over, but it is a very doable and important thing. Salt is the classic way of dealing with it but, as with vitamin A, more immediate things can be done such as providing a capsule of iodine which lasts one or two years, or providing for iodine through drinking water. This can be done in the form of a little silicone-based thing in which iodine slowly comes out and lasts a year or so.

Barbara Underwood: Thank you for these illustrations and for your comments. Some of you may not know about these new developments and may want to talk with Dr. Greaves about them later. We move on to Dr. Judith McGuire of the World Bank.

Judith McGuire: Thank you. I would like to offer commentary in the form of historical background and discuss some exciting new future prospects in the nutrition field. I am honored and pleased to be here. I think it is a momentous occasion not only because of the presentation of startling new findings from India, but also because I think it represents a coming of age of nutrition. This is the first World Food Day program, to my mind, that has focused exclusively on nutrition, acknowledging the crucial role that nutrition plays in solving world hunger. You may recall, World Food Day started at the World Food Conference in 1973 and the context of that meeting was a serious drought in the African Sahel. People at that time were quite concerned about famine. In terms of vitamin A they were concerned about blindness. Iodine deficiency, we thought, had been taken care of, and its only manifestation appeared to be goiter. We thought undernutrition was a protein problem. We were looking for quick technological solutions. Then, as now, aggregate world food supplies were adequate. They are still adequate. This throws the gauntlet down to nutritionists to say the challenge is providing the right quality and quantity of food to all individuals at the appropriate and necessary times in their lives.

Since the 1973 World Food Conference we have had much more extensive documentation of the nutrition problem in developing countries. We know much more about managing drought and famine. The Botswana experience is quite compelling in this regard. We know now it is not necessarily a failure of food supply as much as a failure of purchasing power and access to food which causes famine. We have the findings of Dr. Rahmathullah, and other findings on vitamin A and its effect on morbidity, mortality, and growth. We have come to appreciate the range of effects of iodine deficiency in relation to growth and development, mental development and physical disabilities. We have come up with a new mass-dosage approach for addressing iodine deficiency. We have quantified the effects of iron deficiency not only on productivity, which is its most obvious effect, but also on infection, on learning, and on reproductive outcomes.

In terms of undernutrition, we have much better documentation as a result of a number of studies concerning the effect of undernutrition and chronic undernutrition on morbidity, mortality, cognitive developments, work productivity, and reproductive function. We have come to appreciate the importance of dietary quality. It is no longer perceived as simply a problem of calories and food quantity. We also have made a number of programmatic advances. Growth monitoring and nutrition counseling have come of age, and we have a number of experiences showing that they can work. As you will learn this afternoon, the social marketing of positive health and nutrition behaviors is quite doable and numerous methods exist for influencing behavioral change in the nutrition area.

Fortification, as we learned this morning, has developed far beyond our wildest dreams of years ago. We have new compounds, new vehicles, new techniques. As Peter Greaves just mentioned, we can iodize well water. Doubly fortified salt with iodine and iron is within reach. We have developed slow-release iron preparations. We have mass-dose vitamin A and iodine. In terms of other kinds of nutrition interventions, we also have made advances.

Food stamps targeted to the most vulnerable households have been effectively used in a number of countries. Targeted feeding programs, combined with nutrition education and growth monitoring, as is the case in the Iringa Integrated Nutrition Program in Tanzania, have been shown to be very effective in reducing rates of malnutrition. I should point out that these programs are not only for children who fall below the third degree of malnutrition, but for those children who are growth faltering. New programs provide child care along with feeding and health care for those children whose mothers have to be off at work either seasonally or on a long-term basis. Extending financial credit to women, to women's work cooperatives, combined with nutrition education, appears to be an effective new program at the community level.

We have made much progress, which is evident in the fact that in August 1989 there were two meetings at the International Congress of Nutrition—one organized by the Nutrition Planner's Forum, the other organized by the United Nations Subcommittee on Nutrition—both of which were entitled, "What Works For Nutrition." We have developed a critical mass of effective nutrition programs which can improve nutrition considerably and do so cost effectively and on a sustainable basis.

But there are challenges ahead and I think many people here have spoken of them. There are still an estimated one hundred and forty million children or so who will be experiencing growth failure. There are a billion anemic people in the world, two-thirds of pregnant women are anemic, two hundred million people have iodine deficiency, and several hundred thousand people are severely vitamin A deficient. Over 15 percent of children are born with low birthweight. This suggests to me a great number of women of reproductive age are malnourished, and they are giving birth to low birthweight babies.

Today, we have been provided with various blueprints for addressing these problems, for meeting these challenges. We have the research component, and Dr. Rahmathullah embodies for me the proper spirit of research: research not just for the sake of coming up with a finding, but research for the sake of turning it into action. We have seen innovative applications in the case of iron fortification in China. It takes creativity and innovation to bring the technology into effective programs. We have seen, from Miss Maribe's paper, the importance of training and of institutional development. We know that this is a key link in addressing these problems. We will see this afternoon how social marketing can and should be an integral part of programs that seek to improve health and nutrition. We will learn from Dr. Monckeberg the importance of sustained commitments over the long period which are not tied to any particular political party but which reflect on the importance of political will in supporting health and nutrition programs.

I think political will continues to be a key variable in all of this. We also have seen that what we need is cooperation and commitment. We need this between the research and the operational people, between national and international institutions, between the private food industry, private drug industry, and the public organizations, NGOs, foundations, as well as among the different sectors. It is not just an issue of the health sector; it can also affect agriculture, education, and commerce and foreign trade.

We have seen great progress in the nutrition field, and we need to come out of this meeting with renewed energy and commitment to addressing nutrition and hunger problems. We certainly have the tools. I think a meeting like this shows that there is sufficient motivation, knowledge, and awareness that nutrition is a key component in addressing the world hunger problem.

Barbara Underwood: Thank you both for your comments. Our speakers may want to respond to the comments. I would like to throw out something that spans the concerns at least of two of the speakers. Miss Maribe and Dr. Rahmathullah both brought out the fact that it is important to get communities involved, to enlist community participation in some of these programs. Reflecting on Dr. Rahmathullah's work, as reported in her paper, one can ask, how was it possible on a weekly basis to get to 15,400 children and to have coverage at the level of 88 percent? Dr. Rahmathullah mentioned the importance of the availability of information at the community level and its role in a sustainable program. I wonder if the two of you might want to comment a little further on the issue of community participation and how critical it is and whether you think we can take that into consideration in our national planning, and how this can be done?

Tshire Maribe: My experience in Botswana indicates that since national independence the spirit of what people call self-reliance has tended to die down. This has happened, I think, because the government assumes too much responsibility for ensuring that people's welfare will be taken care of. Traditionally, we had a system in which people did things themselves. They knew that it was part of their responsibility as citizens to do those things themselves. After independence, however, the government began to take that responsibility away from people; I think it is the same reason that accounted for the government intervening so much during the six years of drought. That made people sit back and say to themselves, "Well, somebody else is going to do it for us."

Now, we don't know what can turn the situation back to the past, to the traditional approach of self-reliance. I feel very strongly, nevertheless, that information may be one of the strategies that we will have to employ in Botswana to try to do this. The Botswana system of information, as I indicated, is largely organized from the top down. Yet even though it starts from the national level and flows downward, we have evidence of information being utilized by community leaders, utilized within the context of a traditional setting, to make certain decisions where people are allowed to use this information to come up with effective actions. And when this happens, it allows people to feel as if they came up with the idea, they were involved in its initiation, and then they feel like participants in it.

I think that in Botswana for a very long time to come, there will be a strong interest in utilizing the strategy of getting community-based information to circulate throughout the system simply because it does give people a sense of ownership. And when people feel as though they own something, they always take an interest in wanting to follow it up. This is for me the kind of work and one of the major strategies that has been adopted in Botswana and to a large extent in the ECSA organization.

Barbara Underwood: Thank you. Dr. Rahmathullah, would you like to comment?

V. Rahmathullah: Actually, I find it rather odd that people should ask how we have community participation because I think that is the simplest thing to do. As a research project, what I did was simply to explain that I was doing the research work to try and find out the effect of two vitamins. I did this in very simple language to all the political leaders in the community, to all the franchised union presidents, and to the chairmen of the unions. Secondly, all the staff who were employed to collect the data were drawn from the community while the criterion for the job was that the person had to live in the community. So, by the time the research project was over, we had provided jobs to a large number of families so they were all feeling obligated to comply with our requirement, especially when I said that I didn't know whether the vitamin is good or bad. I think that people understood why there was a need to be honest about what they were reporting to us and why they should take the vitamin supplement without failure. And I think it worked well.

Barbara Underwood: Thank you very much. I see that some of you from the audience would like to make some comments or ask some questions of our speakers.

Questioner: Dr. Rahmathullah, in your presentation you mentioned the failure of India's primary health care system to provide adequate health and nutrition support. It doesn't appear that on a national basis community participation can easily be achieved. I wonder how much of that participation, as seen in your study, is a function of available resources and of very good organizing skills?

Barbara Underwood: I will try to summarize what I think the question is. The national health care program in India, as Dr. Rahmathullah pointed out, is not reaching more than about a third of those who need to be reached—a relatively small proportion of the total. That program is primarily within the health infrastructure. And Dr. Rahmathullah is suggesting it should be more community based. The question is: are the resources there to make it more community based?

V. Rahmathullah: In India the primary health care system has not been integrated with the village-based health worker scheme. We have village health workers, Anganwadi workers, community nutrition workers, and so on. These nutrition workers and the Anganwadi workers are not integrated within the health system. They don't come under the health system. They come under the social welfare board. The health system uses these organizations in order to improve its reach to the public.

117

There is little communication between the community and the primary health care system. The primary health care system seems to be content to work in isolation, without enlisting community involvement. At present, there are a lot of efforts being made to integrate the community health worker into the primary health care system. But in the initial stage of the experiment, it was clear that the community health care workers were recruited through the political system and not by the health care system. So we are experiencing a problem. However, there are a lot of efforts going on to achieve integration. If that integration takes place, then the primary health care system will become more effective. At present, the primary health system is not effective.

Questioner: I'd like to support Dr. Rahmathullah's work and her emphasis on health education, family food production, and the consumption of nutritious foods. These approaches have been questioned in the past. It used to be said that nutrition education does not work. Children in Wisconsin, where I was growing up in 1920s, were by and large not eating vegetables, especially fresh vegetables. They were not drinking milk in the rural areas. So, we got out of the laboratory and went around the state lecturing about the need to have a balanced diet. It was badly needed. The U.S. Department of Agriculture documented that as a result of these educational activities, the consumption of fresh fruits and vegetables rose markedly in the middle and later 1920s.

Also, Dr. Rahmathullah is absolutely correct that many of the earlier efforts in promoting community and family gardens in many countries faltered because they did not receive even minimal support from the agricultural authorities or from anyone else in a position of authority. This support can take the form of providing good quality seeds in some cases and things of that sort. But these things have to be done, and I am glad to say that no longer, as in the case of 1960s, are agriculturalists and economists inclined to ridicule this kind of effort. They are beginning to take health and nutrition much more seriously.

Questioner: Dr. Rahmathullah has pointed out, rightly, that the problem of vitamin A deficiency is serious among children under three years of age. I think many countries have succeeded in promoting community and household vegetable gardens; but the problem we're facing now is that we cannot be sure that these vegetables will be eaten by those who are most in need. How can we be sure that these vegetables will be eaten instead of sold as a crop? Another problem is, how can we get enough of these vegetables with vitamin A to children who are under three years of age, when their parents lack the understanding of the need, or lack access to these foods?

Barbara Underwood: I know in my own experience that if the grownups in the family do not eat their green leafy vegetables, the young children certainly are not going to do it. Part of this whole process of education is to practice what we preach at all levels. Dr. Horwitz?

Abraham Horwitz: At my age one can hardly have a voice. My question is directed to Miss Maribe. I was very impressed with your paper, impressed with the ap-

118

proach—capacity building, institutional strengthening, over the long range. I am glad that in the meantime, efforts are being made in these ten or fifteen countries to develop nutrition interventions based on sound information. My question relates to my position with the United Nations Subcommittee on Nutrition. We are distressed with the situation in Africa and, therefore, we have consulted with the World Health Organization committee on Africa about a resolution endorsing a task force to develop a nutrition plan for the 1990s. The plan has been reviewed, and it was felt that, perhaps, it was too ambitious, too top-down, having very little community participation. You have told us today about a number of countries in Africa working together, that seem to be ecologically, politically, environmentally similar. I understood that there are four regional groups in all. Are they pursuing the same approach? And what would be your advice to us? Should we make a plan for the region as a whole? Or should we follow what groups of countries such as East, Central, and Southern African Food and Nutrition Cooperation (ECSA) are doing?

Tshire Maribe: I am very pleased that you enjoyed my paper. I have had opportunities to present papers at conferences that you chaired, and I think you make a very effective chair. First of all, I have had problems with the constitution of the task force that is developing the concept of a decade for Africa—a food and nutrition decade for Africa. As a matter of fact, we in ECSA are the only subregion that is organized well enough to have a program and a budget and that is talking about having a permanent position of a coordinator. But even with this kind of progress, we are not, you know, a member of this task force. I just don't know how you can then have a program that would cogently address the issues at the basic level of the community. Therefore, I am very pleased that some people have asked that this program be reviewed. I have had an opportunity to discuss the membership of the task force with FAO in Rome and they accept my position. Unfortunately, what has happened is that the other four subregions of Africa have not taken off.

I was discussing this issue the other day with some of my colleagues and I said, maybe it's just as well that we should take a very cautious approach to this. Let ECSA as one of the subregions that has already taken off be an example to the other four subregions. I think it is better to be small and build your strength up than to start big and then have to diminish your strength downward. I'm not disappointed with the fact that things have evolved this way. I am very pleased and I am just hoping that the other subregions will be willing enough to learn from the ECSA experience. I feel that if there is a strategy, an approach, a program, to dedicate a decade to food and nutrition activities, I think that it is best to involve ECSA as much as possible. This will ensure that whatever commitment and decisions are taken can be followed up on because we already have in place the mechanism for following up on issues. Secondly, we would ensure that the strategies we come up with would benefit these countries because we already have drawn up a program of collaboration that our own activities reflect. I think that it would be unnecessary duplication if somebody else comes up with another program that they feel would be useful for the entire African region to take on. My advice would be to ensure that we are free to participate, and secondly to involve us at ECSA.

Barbara Underwood: Are there some other questions from the floor?

Questioner: I have some questions about the vitamin A study. In the October 4 *New York Times,* the headline read: "Childhood Deaths Cut by Half with Vitamin A." So that's a very dramatic statement that the public reads and gets excited about. Obviously it's not the kind of statement that the organized vitamin A community would make. So my question really is, how do we qualify that statement? This particular study was focusing on children in a very high-risk group, with a very high prevalence of vitamin A deficiency, apparently with a very large prevalence of chronic malnutrition. Secondly, I want to pick up on Peter Greaves's comment about megadose distribution. Vitamin A megadose capsule distribution perhaps has moved from a short-term strategy to an ongoing strategy. This leads to the question, what is the future of megadose capsule distribution?

Barbara Underwood: Dr. Rahmathullah, would you like to comment?

V. Rahmathullah: In India, we feel that the megadose approach cannot be left in the hands of nonprofessionals. In the primary health care system, vitamin A distribution through the paramedical people who have handled it has been very poor. This means that we need to find an alternative way of distributing vitamin A. If the megadose cannot be left in the hands of the nonprofessionals, then we have no other choice but to turn to safe dosage levels in the hands of the nonprofessionals. That is why my recommendation was that if we have lower dose vitamin A, it can be safely left with the Anganwadi worker or the village health worker or the nutrition worker who can give it as often as she or he contacts those children.

Barbara Underwood: I might make a brief comment on the first question. If you know how to control the headlines on press releases, please let me know. You do your best to make sure they get the right message but there's just no way you can control what newspapers adopt as their headlines.

I think there is a place for the high dose of vitamin A. Dr. Rahmathullah certainly has stressed that there is no one strategy that universally can be applied in every place. I think that what she was pointing out is that a high-dose supplementation program is something that is probably not sustainable and that it must be coupled with a program that tries to get these long-term strategies in place so that you can phase out the use of high-dose supplements. Now there are places in certain countries where there is no water. There's no way they can grow green leafy vegetables. What water is present they are using to grow wheat, or corn, or the staple of the area. And in those situations it is not practical to think in terms of an educational program to grow green leafy vegetables. Certainly, if you have a vitamin A deficiency problem in such areas, a high-dose capsule is probably an appropriate approach. At least, it is one of the options that should be considered. Certainly, the high dose should be available for treatment.

When you have a child with signs of vitamin A deficiency, giving a high-dose capsule of vitamin A might be appropriate. I'm sure we can think of other situations where that approach might be appropriate. I do not think anyone wants to throw out the high-dose capsule approach. We simply want to have a careful analysis of individual situations within a country and of what resources are available. This involves assessing the magnitude and the severity of the problem and then using good sense in selecting a strategy that is affordable, acceptable, sustainable, and safe.

There is one other point to make. I don't want to close the session before coming back to a point that Dr. Greaves brought out that deals with this question of contact. He said, "Have we got to start to rethink programs that can get us more in contact at the household level?" We professionals in this field have argued a long time about contact effects. And do they explain some of these facts, these findings, that we have above and beyond treatment? If you will excuse me, Dr. Rahmathullah, for talking about it, but the program that she described to us involved a weekly contact. And when she looked at the anthropometric responses of these children to the one year of intervention, she reported she could not show any treatment effect on growth. But we looked at that group of children during that one year interval and broke them down into nutritional status—stunted, wasted, stunted and wasted, the normal children, anthropometrically speaking.

Then we looked at the incremental growth during that one-year period. Remember, we didn't get a treatment effect of vitamin A. But you know, we got a linear response in the stunted children that was much more significant than in any other nutritional category. How do you explain it? If it wasn't a treatment thing, then I think it was a contact effect. I do not think that it was related directly to food intake because we couldn't show that effect on weight. But stunting is a characteristic of deprived households and there are many elements that produce that stunting, of which diet is only one, but not the only one. And it seems to me that in this contact with the most deprived households in these villages, things were changing within that household context that had a positive effect on the children's growth.

Dr. Greaves, I think we are beginning to get some objective evidence, some quantitative figures, on the positive effect of contact. Indeed, we may want in the future to think more and more about how we can really develop contacts at a local level. I think that is the way it is going to have to come, namely, systems that draw out these households of the most deprived people from their isolation and bring them into contact with the community, in order to bring about improvement in health among the most deprived.

Peter Greaves: I am very pleased to hear you say that. I think it is very encouraging and very important. In a phrase, it seems to me that it kind of supports the triad concept I talked about in terms of food, health, and care. And one can make a good case for arguing that the greatest of those is care.

Questioner: One point strikes me as missing which is critical. In terms of contact, in terms of care, in terms of changes of behavior at the household level, in terms of input of information that's going to be useful to nutrition and food planning, we need to genderize people. We need to really be conscious of the different behaviors of men and women, the different roles of men and women, the different statuses.

Of the things we have discovered, anything that increases the status of women in a community almost automatically improves the health of the children in that community. I just want to add a note of caution in our language. We have got to start teaching ourselves not to say, "people," but to say, "men" and "women"; not to say, "heads of households." Women live in households; men live in households. Not just community leaders. Which community leaders? How open was the input of the women in the Indian village communities? How many of those union leaders were women? Where did the women's input come in? I would be very interested if it were possible to do follow-up research on that contact effect. You see, if one of the things that was happening to those deprived households is that the role of the mothers in feeding the children was gaining more status, then that can explain the improvements in child health.

Barbara Underwood: Thank you very much for that very perceptive comment. I could not agree with you more, and how I wish we could go back into those communities and do the kind of studies that you are talking about. We have to ask ourselves continuously: What did we do through that particular nutrition program that changed things within the household? And who changed? There is time for one last question.

Questioner: I guess it is more of a comment than a question. The contact effect is a complicated sociological issue. My only plea would be, as workers walk around the villages and communities contacting people, that they keep the vitamin A in their pocket and take the immunization syringe along and they take it to the household. They also should keep the education analogy in focus and the desire to change attitudes and practices involving child care, maternal care, and nutritional education. We know this works.

Barbara Underwood: Thank you. We have had a very full morning, very fine presentations, and certainly a good discussion. I want to thank all the speakers for their presentations, the commentators, and the audience.

Afternoon Discussion

Norge Jerome: It is a great pleasure to introduce Dr. Abraham Horwitz, a friend of mine who has many titles and a great deal of experience in the health and nutrition fields. I note in this context his role as chair of the International Vitamin A Consultative Group (IVACG) and as chair of the United Nations Subcommittee on Nutrition. Dr. Horwitz will lead off the discussion on the two papers that were presented earlier.

Abraham Horwitz: Thank you very much Dr. Jerome, colleagues, and ladies and gentlemen. Of course, I am very honored to be here but I believe that the organizers made a terrible mistake in selecting me. I am terribly biased in favor of one of the papers because I have known Dr. Monckeberg for a great number of years. I am one of his admirers and he showed today what he has done in one country, in Chile, that, as I am going to say, can be reproduced in other countries in the developing world. Secondly, I am respectfully critical of Dr. Roberto's paper but since this is not my field, I am presenting only my doubts, my reservations. I hope you will forgive me.

Turning to Dr. Monckeberg, he has presented a successful national experience in health and nutrition, in human and social development, according to all indicators. The country has a wealth of reliable data, which when properly analyzed and interpreted, demonstrates the progress that has been made. In Chile information has been used effectively for decision making. The country has reduced mortality, morbidity, malnutrition, and low birthweight, and has increased life expectancy to levels similar to those that characterize a number of industrialized societies. This process has occurred, according to Dr. Monckeberg, in spite of civil and economic crises, economic stagnation, and political upheavals.

The fact is, as Dr. Monckeberg has shown, that Chile has an average life expectancy that is clearly above average in relation to per capita income. It is an example of good health at relatively low cost. Attaining these levels of well-being for the country as a whole has taken three decades. And this is to my mind one of the lessons to be learned from Dr. Monckeberg's presentation and his unremitting efforts. It is important because we are witnessing a series of lofty goals in health and nutrition advanced by United Nations agencies and to be accomplished in the developing world during the 1990s. Significant amounts of extra budgetary funds are being requested. We all hope that they will be forthcoming. International banks have already expressed their willingness to increase their investments in child health and nutrition, and this is certainly encouraging. But even then we should be careful not to promise more than we can deliver, and this message to my mind should go to the national and international communities dealing with food, nutrition, and health.

As Dr. Monckeberg points out, and I quote, "Human resources are the most important elements for social development, and I consider that this is something that has not been sufficiently recognized." To train people according to their respective responsibilities, providing field support, supervising and retraining them, all takes time. This involves more than management as applied to nutrition and health, a distinct discipline and a phase for organizing effective services. There are other lessons to be learned.

In dealing with government, Dr. Monckeberg claims that it is essential to be a leader and have credibility based mainly on scientific prestige, together with flexibility, persistence, and patience. This is, of course, his personal experience and perhaps the model cannot always be duplicated. However, the need to ensure that political decisions are based on the best scientific evidence available and implemented by applying proven technologies and developing well-managed programs is essential. This is the responsibility of food, nutrition, and health scientists in active dialogue with the decision makers. We realize that in some cases the prevailing political ideologies have interfered with this rational approach. We are advised by Dr. Monckeberg to influence political decision making by creating a consciousness of the consequences of malnutrition and ill health for economic and social development. We are also advised to facilitate health and nutrition programs within the context of the socioeconomic strategy of the government. And most important, he advises practitioners to keep their independence from the political process so as to be able to retain credibility and ensure that specific programs will be sustained, regardless of changes in administration. All in all, it is not a small order of business.

An unsuccessful experience led Dr. Monckeberg to conclude that a large-scale nutrition policy is an impossible dream and perhaps it is not necessary. Thereafter, he told us, efforts in Chile were concentrated fundamentally in those specific interventions for improving the nutritional status of target groups. I have the impression that the failure was not any nutrition policy engineered by Dr. Monckeberg, but rather the nutrition planning process to implement it. This was multisectoral, including all components of the food chain and the myriad of variables therein, with everything depending on everything else. Models were too complex to be understood by the decision makers and very difficult to manage. Nutrition policy and nutrition planning became discredited.

Now, the United Nations Subcommittee on Nutrition is reviewing the issues related to nutrition policies and policies relevant to better nutrition. On the basis of the experience of the 1980s, it is considering nutrition as a series of outcomes. Nutrition planning is still relevant though it should focus on a range of policies and induce actions to reduce malnutrition as a principal outcome.

Another important lesson learned from the Chilean experience is that investments and actions are necessary in order to transfer national income to the people through social services. No single action can explain the outcomes; rather, it is a cluster of things, within several specific sectors, developed concurrently with interventions from other sectors. This includes, Dr. Monckeberg showed us, primary and secondary education, especially of women; food supplementation; water supplies; waste disposal; personal hygiene; health education; and family planning. These interventions are synergistic and together have contributed significantly to reduce morbidity and mortality rates.

Dr. Monckeberg also has discussed ways to improve the effectiveness and efficiency of the health care system. He showed us a number of reforms. The organization of a national basic health care infrastructure is, for the author, the first step in implementing a nutrition and health policy. In Chile this health system has been developed from top to bottom with different levels of complexity for the performance of preventive and curative actions.

I remember distinctly that in my time, thirty-five years ago, we did not even talk about the community or community involvement because we did not think it was necessary to consider the people when we were going to provide them with what was good for them. Times have shown that it doesn't work that way. It is the system as the whole that ensures coverage through effective referrals of patients. At the community level, particularly in the rural area, health units have to reach out to the homes to identify the sick and malnourished, refer them when necessary, educate families, and collect data.

According to Dr. Monckeberg, and I quote him, "The personnel has developed an attitude of service and commitment to the community, whose respect they have gained. In turn, the population has been made aware of its rights and responsibilities in relation to health." Thus, some degree of social consciousness exists in Chile today, stemming from the interpretation of life and the value ascribed to the health and nutrition of mothers and children.

The Chilean experience shows, however, that there has not been a single integrated plan. Nor have specific programs been implemented in all sociographic areas. What explains the differentials between and within them? Activities from different sectors have proceeded simultaneously, reflecting a synergism among them. It could be asked whether the experience of Chile, so clearly explained by Dr. Monckeberg, is relevant to other developing countries in the Americas and in other regions of the world? I am inclined to believe that for similar health and nutrition problems the Chilean approach could be adapted to the culture and to the environmental circumstances of other societies. In fact, during the period discussed in Dr. Monckeberg's paper a number of countries of the Americas have reached comparable levels of progress. Others in the same or in different regions could follow through. The scientific, technical, and operational bases are evident.

Much will depend on sustained political will and commitment to social equity and the response of the people to the opportunity to contribute to health and human betterment. It also will depend on the nature and extent of the problem, and on the quality and quantity of resources available for dealing with the problem, and on the investments from foreign governments and from the community. It is noteworthy that the whole process of health improvement in Chile was accomplished in a period when loans were not available and when grants were very difficult to obtain. With a few exceptions that Dr. Monckeberg referred to, in general, a large extent of the progress has been made entirely with national resources. I believe a government, any government, has to be careful in taking international loans without thinking ahead. After all, what are they going to do when external assistance ends?

The organizers of the colloquium should be commended for having given Dr. Monckeberg the opportunity to describe Chile's success in progressively improving the health and nutrition of the people, an endeavor in which he played such an outstanding role.

Now, if you allow me two or three minutes more. I wrote some comments on Dr. Roberto's social marketing paper, which I studied very carefully.

Promoting appropriate knowledge, attitudes, and practices for better health and nutrition has become a distinct discipline. It has given scientific, technological, and operational bases to health and nutrition education. This process is the result of the biological and social sciences focussing on specific conditions and targeting the groups at higher risk of ill health and malnutrition.

Because the pace of formal education and cultural imitation as well as economic development has been too slow to induce better health, the need to address people directly and call their attention to the consequences of their behavior has become urgent. Mothers as agents of significant change are our main target related to acute diseases of children. However, society as a whole must be included in any condition that affects large groups of human beings requiring a healthier life style.

The present circumstances of the world are not encouraging to predict an increase in the pace of economic development, formal education, and social mobility, and to reduce poverty. Furthermore, population pressures militate against these goals. Although in some countries the rate of increase of the malnourished has diminished, their total numbers have increased. Again, to enlist the informed cooperation of target groups in a population becomes an essential and efficient resource, highly cost effective.

I submit that perhaps the greatest contribution of the Primary Health Care movement—the integrated and not the selective one—has been the opportunity for the active participation of the people in the decisions that deal with their health and nutritional status, as well as involving their families and the communities where they live. But this fundamental objective cannot and will not be reached through the traditional health and nutrition education approaches. Experience shows that these traditional methods did not sufficiently motivate people, because messages were not understood and the need for changing behaviors deleterious to health was not felt.

Because of the lack of proper information, mothers still unknowingly infect their children with acute conditions, e.g., diarrheal disease; adults infect each other with AIDS; and people, in general, regardless of size of income, reduce their life expectancies through diets that tax their cardiovascular system and perhaps induce cancer. There is no need to mention the series of addictions that severely impair health and increase mortality rates. These patients need understanding, treatment, and advice as to how to get rid of these banes.

There is, therefore, an urgent need to inform the people of the risks they face if they do not change their behavior to prevent disease and promote health. This must be, per force, an iterative process that uses specific messages, culturally based, and well-defined communication technologies with a highly scientific content. The social and biological sciences, ideally properly integrated, have the major role to play.

I am impressed with what Dr. Roberto has done in his field. To my mind, one of the greatest breakthroughs in the field of health and nutrition in the last ten or fifteen years has been to transform routine nutritional health education into an undertaking that is scientifically based, reflecting the research accomplishments of the biological and the social sciences. I am inclined to speak of nutrition and of

126

health education as closely connected. This is for me an important breakthrough, especially in view of the slow place of economic development.

Changing the behavior of people, for me, has become fundamental. It may turn out to be the most cost-effective of the health and nutrition measures. So I am all for the process. But I have some doubts. I say that Dr. Roberto has made an important contribution in this field with his paper. He focuses on the implementation of nutrition programs, a phase which is usually underestimated. He quotes Dr. Alan Berg of the World Bank who says that implementation is often neglected. Dr. Roberto considers social marketing a management practice, a discipline of implementation. His approach is pragmatic. We have heard some of the anecdotes he has told us. It is a discipline that uses a systemic approach to communications, leading to changes in behavior as indicated.

But I have the impression that Dr. Roberto's model uses a terminology and a methodology that are closer to those employed in commercial marketing. The emphasis is on product, place, promotion, and price. Each one involves distinct market tools: advertising, adoption promotion, distribution placement, service delivery, cost management and pricing, and a mix of them. They are to be applied successively and conveniently until committed adoption is reached. The process, according to Dr. Roberto, reflects the hounding of adopter behavior, pursuing adopters relentlessly until the victim succumbs. The approach is to pursue the target groups relentlessly, unyieldingly, until the target adopters eventually and finally succumb. No wonder that social marketing has been labeled manipulative. Often, according to Dr. Roberto, and I quote, "It is feared because it may work." Personally, I doubt that this could be considered a scientific approach to promote better health and nutrition.

In the paper we are told what to do in order to change behaviors related to specific health and nutrition issues, but not how to do it. Dr. Roberto does not refer to the method used to get doctors, for example, to respond as expected to the social marketing tools. Modern nutrition education applies methodologies strongly based on the social sciences. They are systematic and carefully structured from qualitative, formative research to quantitative evaluation. The methodology goes through a series of phases that ensure that the target adopter receives specific messages to promote changes in his or her attitudes and practices. The field as a whole appears to have over-emphasized audience effects, particularly through mass media messages, while underemphasizing institutionalization. If we really want developing countries to become self-reliant and self-sufficient in this fundamental field, we should strengthen the process of institutionalization and at the same time continue applying effective methodologies to induce better health and nutrition practices.

For this purpose, I wonder whether we need to apply or adopt the principles and methods of commercial marketing. What we want is to persuade people and not to lose them. Once convinced and properly informed, we expect them to actively change their behavior so as to avert death, prevent disease and malnutrition, and promote health. The biological and the social sciences have designed appropriate methodologies and should, through research, create even more efficient and cost-effective programs. Furthermore, some may question the ethics of the tools of commercial marketing; for instance, profit and advertising. That certainly does not fit with the ideals that nutrition and health education pursue. Thank you.

Norge Jerome: Thank you very much for your comments, Dr. Horwitz. I am sure Dr. Roberto is anxious to respond but if you will bear with us, your time will come, because we would like to hear next from Dr. David Yeung. Dr. Yeung is a professor at Mahidol University in Thailand, at several institutions in the People's Republic of China, and in Canada. Dr. Yeung.

David Yeung: Thank you, Dr. Jerome. My experience in Asian development is limited to my involvement in China and in Thailand in recent years, as head of the Heinz Institute of Nutritional Sciences. My comments this afternoon will therefore be directed to my experience in China and a little bit about Thailand as well.

There is no doubt that to effect sustainable changes in attitudes and behaviors related to health demands a multitude of strategies that are appropriate to the culture, education, and economic conditions of the target population. Social marketing is but one of the strategies that has proven to be effective in certain situations. We do not have to look too far for examples of its effectiveness. In Canada and in the United States, social marketing has been instrumental in raising awareness in the population of the health hazards associated with smoking. However, it is only through the integration of social marketing with the other strategies that the desired behavior change is brought about. For example, the decline in cigarette smoking is brought about not only by the increased awareness of the health hazards of smoking but also by a policy change in legislation that restricts smoking in public places while at the same raising the price of cigarettes. Other factors are personal education and societal pressure to stop smoking, and the environmental changes which facilitate smoking cessation so that making the right choice is the easy choice.

There are other public health examples, particularly in developing countries, in which social marketing together with other strategies has been successful in community development and in encouraging decision making at the grass roots level. The Chilean experience, so eloquently described by Dr. Monckeberg in his paper, is another example of the efficacy of an integrated approach to improving national health and nutrition.

According to Dr. Roberto, I quote, "To get the impressive gains from past nutritional research, policy development, planning and policy formulation directed to the targeted beneficiaries, the malnourished, we now need to attend to the program management skills and process management." I totally agree with this statement. Improvement in management skills at the levels from headquarters to field operations is one of the key elements to success.

Today's business attitude is quality management. There is a commitment to involvement of all people in the process, to continually search for improvement in the quality of service and goods delivered so that total satisfaction of the customers can be achieved. Otherwise, loss of market share and profit will result. Such a commitment recognizes the importance of a complete understanding of the customer's requirements; of aligning resources in systems with strategic plans; executing strategic plans in a methodical way; removing barriers that negatively affect performance, leadership, and teamwork; and to ensure that everyone in the process is responsible for quality. Thus, quality management, together with the right implementation strategy, the right marketing mixes that are appropriate to the culture and the economy, the backing by the right government departments, adequate financing and resources—all of this will likely increase the prospects for the desired behavioral change. This also recognizes that behavior change is profoundly influenced by the political, social, economic, and physical environments in which people live. Nevertheless, the concept of quality management needs to be instilled in all health and nutrition programs. This is our biggest challenge in the People's Republic of China in our effort to upgrade nutrition skills. Let me quickly explain the situation. When the H. J. Heinz company first considered business in China, market research indicated that nutritious and safe baby foods were in short supply despite the vast improvement in the economy and in food distribution. Furthermore, the research revealed that there was a great desire for modern and scientific information on infant nutrition and feeding. Heinz decided to build a modern factory in south China to manufacture affordable nutritionally fortified infant cereals that could be used to combat the prevalent nutrition problems such as iron deficiency, as described so ably by Dr. Liu this morning.

At the same time, we decided to take initiatives to assist China in strengthening its scientific base for nutrition and for safety. The latter began by conducting qualitative research with health professionals, educators, and academics. The research revealed that the priorities should be to assist in strengthening the nutrition knowledge of pediatricians, nutritionists, and public health professionals who would, with their scientific skills and knowledge, better perform their duties. Consequently, the Heinz Institute of Nutritional Sciences was founded. An advisory council, consisting of twenty prominent Chinese nutritionists and pediatricians from different parts of China and three consultants from the United States and Canada, was established to guide the activities of the Institute. The program was established in 1986.

In keeping with Dr. Roberto's lecture, I will talk about this program in the framework of social marketing, in terms of how its so-called products and services are themselves marketed to achieve maximum value. The objective of the program is to strengthen the human resources in nutrition with the hope that the professionals and the workers will contribute to nutrition and food security. One activity is an education program that includes an annual international symposium which provides a forum for foreign and local scientists to share their knowledge and exchange ideas about a specific theme dealing with infant nutrition. A second is the publication of the symposium proceedings to capture a wider audience. A third activity is the publication of a quarterly newsletter containing abstracts from international journals to inform scientists in China about current knowledge on infant nutrition. A fourth consists of academic exchanges among nutrition departments in the People's Republic of China, the United States, and Canada through which Chinese nutritionists receive training in Canada and North American nutritionists lecture in China.

The Heinz program is basically free to the target consumers. However, there is a registration fee and a cost to attend the symposium which is held in a different part of China each year. Beyond this, there is only a time investment in terms of assimilating the printed materials and other information on studying abroad. The academic exchange programs are funded by the Canadian government and through grants from Tufts University. Participants in the program receive the latest printed information on nutrition by mail or verbally by attending the symposium. Of course, if training is involved, the individuals receive it at universities either in China or Canada. Promotion of the Institute's products is done through the products themselves and by word of mouth. Basically, the product sells itself. Occasionally, it is done through announcements in health magazines. There appears to be some success in what we have done in the past five years. This is indicated by the quality of infant nutrition information appearing in leading newspapers and in food magazines; the better quality of research the Heinz Institute of Nutritional Sciences supports; and the quality of the articles appearing in local and international journals.

An example of progress in research is the investigation of the growth patterns of infants and the underlying causes of inferior as well as superior growth. Since our last symposium held in 1989, of which the theme was growth and development of Chinese infants in different parts of the world, a project on this subject has been initiated by professors of nutrition in the West China University of Medical Sciences in Chengdu. This is the first time such a study has been conducted in China. Of course, not all the changes, or positive changes, in nutritional sciences can be credited to the Institute since there are other multinationals cooperating in nutrition projects in various parts of China. But I strongly believe that the Heinz Institute of Nutritional Sciences does exert some direct influence on the scientists who have close contacts with the Institute.

Let me now briefly describe the management problems that I alluded to earlier. China has been strictly ruled from the top since the present government came to power about forty years ago. During the cultural revolution, nutritional science was discredited. Nutritionists were assigned to manual labor in the countryside. These experiences have made people complacent and reluctant to accept responsibilities and take risks. Currently, in the various universities in China that I have visited, most of the nutritionists are conducting research limited to areas such as the prevalence of iron deficiency, of zinc deficiency, and of vitamin D deficiency in the growth of Chinese infants. This appears to stem from the priority the central authorities have placed on infant nutrition since the establishment of the one family, one child policy. This also reflects the security of doing research that is popular, perceived to be politically expedient, and uncomplicated because it requires little innovation. This is, in a sense, toeing the line. Therefore, there is a great need to develop management skills and to foster behavior that stresses leadership, acceptance of responsibilities, and boldness to take risks.

China is but one example of a global revolution that is taking place. The challenge of quality management has become more and more an integral part of promoting health, of promoting changes in attitudes and behaviors. We need to establish cadres of knowledgeable individuals in these countries who will lead, champion causes, manage, take risks, and persevere. It is apparent that I am supportive of Dr. Roberto's suggestion that the management and implementation of health programs are vital to achieving positive behavior changes in health and nutrition. Finally, I would like to add that our effort in China and, indeed, in Thailand as well, is an example of the fact that food companies can independently and objectively play an active role in promoting health, in changing health attitudes and behaviors in countries where they operate. Indeed, many large multinational companies are contributing to development. This contribution is only one of the many strategies that are needed to improve nutrition and food security in Asia, Africa, and Latin America.

Norge Jerome: It is very clear that an overriding theme of the day has been the effectiveness of forming partnerships and I think that your commentary bears that out very well. If we are going to achieve the goals that we have set for ourselves in combatting malnutrition, partnerships among industry, academia, and the providers will have to be effectively implemented. We do want to offer some time to Dr. Roberto as well as to Dr. Monckeberg, to respond to the commentaries. I know that Dr. Roberto does want to respond to Dr. Horwitz.

Eduardo Roberto: Thank you very much. I want to assure Dr. Horwitz that I was not offended.

Abraham Horwitz: Thank you.

Eduardo Roberto: Since 1975, my entry into social and development programs has received more negative response than positive, so I am quite used to the criticisms that have legitimately been made. But I want to respond to a number of points that Dr. Horwitz mentioned. First, the idea of social marketing's down-playing of institutionalization.

That has been a concern that the donor agencies that have sponsored my work in this area have expressed and I respond by saying that institution building is a tall order. The only solid contribution I can make is what I call a transfer of technology. So, in every engagement that I have had, I ask for a second person from the agency, such as a ministry of health or a family planning board, who has a reasonable expectation of being retained within the agency to continue the kind of discipline that I represent. I have never really sold social marketing, and the purpose of my participation here is not to do that. I have refused to sell it.

I have come to realize that one cannot help anybody who thinks that he does not need the help. And if someone in an agency, for example, says that he or she has a better way of implementing and managing other than social marketing, then I can respect that. I am the last person to say that I will be able to help. I am only involved in situations when the request for help is initiated by those who need it. So, in terms of institutionalization I have not gone beyond transfer of technology and of the discipline. Of course, I can go into the details of what I mean by a discipline but this is probably not the forum for that.

The other issue that was raised concerns the very ethics of the practice of social marketing. It is too bad that I have only a few minutes to offer a response, but the ethics of social marketing has been a concern of mine not only because of my own background—I came from economics—but also because my own children have questioned my discipline. So in the book that I have written on social marketing, I insisted with my coauthor that I would take charge of the last chapter, that has to do with the ethics of social marketing. It is an involved subject and I do not think I would do justice to it at this time.

The third item that Dr. Horwitz had mentioned concerns the specifics of the "how to" aspect of social marketing. Now, given the choice in this colloquium between describing such specifics and trying to communicate an awareness of what the technique and approach is all about, I chose the latter—to illustrate what it is all about instead of getting into the details of the specifics. So, that was a choice; maybe it was an ill-advised choice that I have made.

Finally, what about the scientific underpinning of bringing about behavioral change? My training is in marketing research; that is where I specialize and that is what I do, for example, in my country right now. It is based on what I believe is a scientific method. And finally, as Dr. Horwitz was talking, I said to myself, "You know, a more disturbing question is, in fact, what is the record of social marketing in helping nutrition policy and programs?"

Norge Jerome: Thank you. Any questions or comments?

Alan Berg: I share in Dr. Horwitz's admiration for the achievements of Dr. Monckeberg, so much so that at this very moment we have a team in Chile looking at the experience and trying to see what might be applicable in other countries. I must confess, however, one small concern on which I welcome your counsel, your advice, in terms of trying to capture that experience in other countries. This has to do with the potentially nutritionally deleterious effects of milk distribution, and the effect it has had on breast-feeding.

Now, going way back, my recollection is that the breast-feeding practices in Chile had plummeted something like 25 percent, going back forty years. My recollection is that Dr. Monckeberg even attributed some of that to the distribution of milk. Well, I know you have had conscious programs to provide incentives and to encourage breast-feeding. But in looking at the numbers in your paper, I'm still a little concerned. You have said you have gone from 25 percent up to 52 percent, which is certainly an accomplishment; but that 52 percent is breast-feeding at three months, as compared to what had been earlier an 85 percent ratio of breast-feeding over a period of six months. I am just concerned, particularly about other countries where the health infrastructure is not nearly as good as Chile's, where they don't have the marketing and nutrition education possibilities that you have in Chile, where they're trying to emulate this extensive milk distribution program which might have these negative effects. I really am seeking your guidance on this, how to get around this, whether there is some product other than milk that might be provided and serve the same purpose, and so on. Thank you.

Fernando Monckeberg: I think that you are perfectly right when you get worried about breast-feeding in relation to wide-scale milk distribution. But again, I want to recall how it happened, and I'm going back thirty years. Thirty years ago, in Chile, most of the mothers used to give breast milk. And most of them used to feed their child by breast. Nevertheless, during those days infant mortality used to be two hundred per thousand. And most of this occurred during the first and second year of life, before any intervention was started. This was the reality.

What has happened in thirty years? Obviously, breast-feeding declined during the time that milk was being distributed. Later on, we started the program to stimulate breast-feeding and again the practice starts to rise, but, nevertheless, it never rises to the earlier level. But infant mortality declined to 17 per thousand. In other words, if our goal was to preserve breast-feeding, we did a very poor job. But if our goal was to prevent malnutrition, we did a very good job. That is something that you have to consider.

What is the real interest? Breast-feeding per se, or prevention of malnutrition? And you have to combine those two factors. Again, I feel that the program of free distribution of milk, without control, through a deficient structure, and without any other type of intervention, has to be very dangerous. But if you do the milk distribution alongside other interventions, then you can have the kind of result that we have had. I do not know if I answered your question.

Questioner: I'm not rising to discuss the Chilean experience. In the light of certain comments about economists, I thought as an economist I could rise, not with a defense, but with an explanation. In actual fact, economists have studied the history of health, and of populations and of demographics, its influence on life expectancy, and so on. Secondly, there is a problem which is arising in a number of countries, for example, in China, that the development of health has exceeded rates of economic growth and this is moving into a technological pattern in which the cheap methods of reducing mortality and improving health no longer are the important ones, as we move to deal with cancer problems, circulatory problems, and such. The latter involves a very expensive technology, assuming we have the necessary technology at all. On another point. Studies of the relation of mortality and GNP showed, among other things, that Cuba and Sri Lanka, for example, are exceptions, statistically speaking. The point I want to make is that they were exceptions twenty years ago, and to explain why they are not in terms of the history of the last thirty or forty years may lead to some miscalculations, about causes and effects of policies.

One final point, if I may. There's a fair amount of research which has indicated that the appropriate policies vary with the stages of development of countries; and by the knowledge and the technologies which may be available to them. Generalizing about all developing countries may not be the most profitable way to find out what's going on.

Norge Jerome: Thank you for your helpful comments.

Peter Greaves: Two brief questions, one to Dr. Monckeberg, one to Dr. Roberto. Dr. Monckeberg, looking at the broad sweep of this historical period, would you argue that the attempt to increase public awareness about these programs was a strategically important factor in taking the actions that were helpful and necessary? That's my question to you. My question to Dr. Roberto is: Could you explain further your statement that it has been shown that focus group discussion is useful in generating ideas for more or better message executions but not for ideas about the better message?

Fernando Monckeberg: As I explained in my paper, the first condition in stimulating a nutrition or health policy is a positive decision at the political level, and this support at the political level has to be induced. And for this you have to use any kind of mass medium communication. Almost every day we use the newspaper, the journals, television, the universities. We trained journalists about nutrition and health. We have trained almost twenty of them and this is extremely important. The other factor is to talk with the politicians directly. When you create an awareness of health and nutrition by means of mass medium communications, then you have arrived at the second step to talk with the politicians. Some of them are fighting to reach power and others are trying to keep power. And you have to translate the benefit of health and nutrition for each politician's ends to reach or maintain power.

During an election time is the most effective period to win support. The last time that we had presidential elections, there were three candidates. One on the left, a second from the right, and the third from the center. For all three of them we prepared a communication program dealing with nutrition and health policy, each with a different modification. During the last election, again we did the same. Each candidate was persuaded to make health and nutrition policy and programs his first priority. Perhaps they didn't know that but in our Institute we have people who represent the different political tendencies, and we exchange and adapt information for this purpose. You are right that once the politician puts nutrition and health on his own agenda, then you can be quite sure that the solution will come.

Norge Jerome: Thank you for your comment. Dr. Roberto?

Eduardo Roberto: The comment on the focus group discussion was triggered by the experience both in the social marketing area and in the commercial marketing area. Let me just show you very quickly the result of the focus group discussion and then what was done. For the condom-marketing campaign, there were a series of mass media communications targeted toward members of families. They were asked if they decided to plan their family and so on, and if they had their way, would they wait for a few more years for their next baby. Then there was a communication addressed to the mother: "If you had your way, wouldn't you wait a few more years for your next baby?" And then a communication in a dialect addressed to the lower class. Now, these came out as the result of the findings of the focus group discussion.

In the focus group discussion what we got was predominantly a reading of the sentiment of the potential adopters of condoms, who expressed that their biggest concern is that it interferes with sexual pleasure. So we said, well, we should address that. The experience with the focus group discussion showed us that a problem exists insofar as people have a way of riding on the bandwagon opinion in the group. A self-appointed leader in the group can persuade the rest of the members in the group to voice the same kind of concern. We were running eight groups. And out of the eight groups, I remember six of them expressed that sentiment that condoms interfere with sexual pleasure.

What we did was basically to quantify it. And let's see what is the best predictor of the attitude and intention to use the condom among the potential adopters. And if it is true that there is a concern about sexual pleasure, then the regression coefficient of that variable, when measured in the survey, should come out as the dominant independent variable. But it did not. What came out instead was the concern about one's responsibility for the family. That has been replicated in my own experience in the business sector. That's the basis of the comment.

Norge Jerome: Thank you very much. I would like Dr. Monckeberg to comment on a statement made by Tshire Maribe this morning, about coordination versus implementation. If you recall, she thought that it was much more successful to have the coordinating group separate from the implementation group. And it seems to me that from your paper, you have had a similar experience. Would you endorse that? The answer, I see you are affirming, is a simple "yes." The coordinating councils then should be located, for example, in a ministry of planning or in a national nutrition council, so they would definitely be separate from an implementation group located in the various ministries.

Questioner: It seems to me that it is not just the separation but the level of the power. The coordinating group has to have the power to carry out actions.

Norge Jerome: Yes, but I think it is more than that. In the Malawi experience, the coordinating group is within the ministry, in the president's office. There are other situations where there are national nutrition councils, perhaps appointed by the president, maybe appointed by various ministers, that are separate from the office of planning or from the president's office. So we're talking about two separate entities with almost equal power, shall we say, but at least they are separate entities. And, yes, power is a real issue. The separation between implementation and coordination, I think, is a major issue that Miss Maribe was bringing forth and it seems to have been an issue in the Chilean experience.

My question to Dr. Roberto deals with applying social marketing to policy makers and to providers. My notion of social marketing is now slightly different. I come from a nutritional anthropology background and I see the involvement with the potential adopter as the means of gathering very important information so that one could reflect it back in communications, in a message, coming from the technical or program group. So it is a sort of melding of the two. Now, we also have to change our behaviors in relation to policy makers and to provider groups. How does one apply these techniques and strategies to the provider group?

Eduardo Roberto: One of the important lessons that we have gained in helping out in development and social programs is the fact that if we just start going after the individual adopters, the end-use beneficiaries, it will take a long time for the objectives to be reached. What stands between the program and the ultimate adopters are really what we call influence groups—the policy makers, those who coordinate the work of the agencies and the implementing of programs. And to me, there is a need for a separate program to reach each one of the influence groups. The idea is really to identify the allies of the program who are in effect then the potential owners of the program. And the objective is very simple: to win the active support of the allies, not just their passive support; and in terms of the opponents, to neutralize them. I agree that a basic issue in this case is power.

Let me take this a step further. To me, the major problem is how to retain the integrity of the program that exists at the headquarters level, and translate it down to the field level. We know that there is a long distance in between the program at the headquarters level and down at the field level. And if we are now talking, let's say, of a coordinating agency, I think what is clearly important is that there must be a separation.

But more than that, I think, is the need for representation of the different bodies that we're talking about. For example, at the field level, it is your extension workers, or midwives, or nurses, who are in charge of implementing the nutrition or health program. And, on top of them is the district and on top of the district is the region and on top of the region is the national headquarters. Now, when you have a headquarters program, it is very rare that the program will retain its integrity when it filters down to the field level. That is because when you get down to the field level, for example, you will find that what is going to be implemented is what the doctor at the health center wants implemented. I have seen this happen. For example, a doctor who is infatuated with vasectomy. Suddenly, in that particular area, vasectomy went up. But it's not the official program. The policy of the government is that we have to have equality for all.

So, by representation I mean that you will have to come down to the fact that you must take account of local and territorial variation. So, if, at the implementation stage, it will come to that, the idea is for the field workers and the supervisors of the field workers to have representation at the planning stage, even in the coordination process.

It is an old management dilemma. Do you plan quickly by not taking account of field variations and then implement for a long time, or do you plan over an extended period of time but build consensus from those who will actually implement the program? My bias is, of course, the second choice. Take a long time to plan, then you can build consensus. Then the variations at the field level will be accounted for, and this process probably will consume the same period of time anyway.

Norge Jerome: Thank you very much, Dr. Roberto, Dr. Monckeberg, Dr. Horwitz, and Dr. Yeung for your participation. This has been an exciting afternoon.

CHAPTER 10

Research Directions in Nutrition and Food Security: Proceedings of a Discussion at the International Life Sciences Institute-North America

Timothy Morck: I would like to welcome you to the International Life Sciences Institute-North America on behalf of Dr. Alex Malaspina, president of ILSI-North America. He expresses his wishes for the success of our discussion and looks forward to reading the published proceedings. This roundtable discussion provides an opportunity to explore some of the questions that were raised in our colloquium yesterday; to synthesize the different perspectives; give some guidance to future research needs; perhaps make recommendations. I know Neil Kotler has a couple of comments.

Neil Kotler: It is a pleasure to welcome you. Our aim is to publish today's roundtable discussion, which will form the last section of the colloquium volume jointly developed by the Smithsonian Institution and the International Life Sciences Institute-North America. This will be the fourth volume in the series of publications in conjunction with the awarding of the World Food Prize. Today's discussion presents an excellent opportunity to reexamine the relationship of research, policy, and programs and to bring together the comparative perspectives of several disciplines and the experiences of three continents.

Timothy Morck: Yesterday, we heard a number of key words that kept surfacing: action, implementation, empowerment, integration, and interdisciplinary. One of

---

Editor's Note: In cooperation with the Smithsonian Institution, the International Life Sciences Institute-North America (ILSI-North America) hosted a two-hour roundtable discussion on the morning following the 17 October 1991 colloquium to examine the research and policy implications of the colloquium proceedings. The discussion was taped, transcribed, and edited for publication. In addition to the colloquium speakers, commentators, and moderators, the participants also included Robert F. Chandler, Jr., the 1988 World Food Prize laureate; Samuel G. Kahn of the Office of Nutrition, US AID; and Shubh Kumar of the International Food Policy Research Institute.

the goals today is to explore some of these ideas more fully than we had time to do yesterday.

Dr. Rahmathullah, in her excellent paper, described the ways that India is addressing the vitamin A-deficiency problem. One of these has to do with the efforts to involve agriculturists to a greater degree in home gardening programs and other nutrition and health initiatives. Yet she indicated that this has not been entirely successful up to now.

One of the topics that I would like us to consider this morning are the actions that could be taken in facilitating the interaction and the cross-fertilization between the health and agricultural fields. This may involve research or marketing. This may involve interdisciplinary approaches.

Dr. Liu discussed the conditions of iron deficiency in the People's Republic of China and gave some very interesting and encouraging data from her research trials, showing that fortification has been successful in several forms: in soft drink powders and in soy sauce, as examples. We need to think about how to take this information to the next step; how to put it into action in addressing the great nutritional needs that exist in China and in other countries; and what are the steps necessary to convert the research into effective implementation in local and national programs.

It is unfortunate that Miss Maribe is not able to be with us today. She had a very tight travel schedule that required her early departure yesterday. However, I think we should take the opportunity to discuss further the topic of food security in Africa. I know that Dr. Greaves probably did not have enough time yesterday to air all of his thoughts on this subject. So, this will be an opportunity to follow up on some of those ideas that were not fully explored yesterday.

The pivotal role of women in nutrition and agriculture was mentioned in several papers, in particular, the need to look at the status of women, identify their multiple roles, and find ways to strengthen their position. I think this is a theme that runs throughout the literature on economic development and this is another area that can be explored further.

Dr. Yeung shared his experience with one of the major international food companies and its institution-building initiatives in Asia. I think this avenue deserves investigation and exploration in greater detail, specifically, the business aspects of nutrition and the partnerships between corporations and governments in helping countries solve their health and nutrition problems.

I am extremely interested in giving Dr. Roberto a little more opportunity to share his thinking on specific linkages between nutrition research and policy, on the one hand, and social marketing, on the other. Picking up on one of the questions raised yesterday: how do you effectively take social marketing to the policy makers? How do you influence decision makers to integrate nutrition policy and nutrition programs? There also will be further opportunities to examine the remarkable programs that Dr. Monckeberg helped to create in Chile, and the possibilities for replicating them in other countries. These are action-oriented questions, and I think we have opportunities to address them. These are just a few thoughts that I have. No doubt you may have some others.

I would like to open the discussion with Dr. Rahmathullah. I would like to ask her a little more about the ability to bridge the gap between agriculture and home gardening in India that she described in her paper. What are the impediments you see to this process becoming more effective?

V. Rahmathullah: Actually, the process has already started. In all of the major cities, the horticultural departments are creating programs to encourage home or kitchen gardens of vegetables, mainly for sale in the urban market. These programs should spread to the rural areas, so that more vegetables can be made available there, where the need is great.

Home gardening is also a source of income for poor families. The woman is the one who looks after the kitchen garden; the man is the laborer. She uses her kitchen waste water for her gardening and in growing vegetables, and she can earn some money doing that.

Secondly, the market would have more vegetables available for people to consume. Once more vegetables are available, you will find people eating more vegetables. I have suggested that households should concentrate on growing vitamin A-rich foods.

Timothy Morck: Who do you see as the impetus behind this process?

V. Rahmathullah: Actually, the agricultural department in India has been doing it. As I said, the horticultural department has not been as aggressive in this area as the agricultural department. They currently look out after the cash crops, but they have made a beginning. I think they need a push from people like us, asking them to get more involved in our projects. This would probably give them the impetus to expand support for home gardening.

Timothy Morck: That is a key that I am looking for: who are the people who can move the process along?

Norge Jerome: Yes. I would like to share a success story along these lines. The ivy gourd has been successfully marketed through a social marketing program in northeast Thailand supported by our office. It is a program that brings together a number of sectors, including the ministries of agriculture, of education, of planning, and the ministry of health. They have successfully come together in a community development program to market the ivy gourd, which had not been used traditionally.

Growth of the ivy in the past occurred on tops of houses and was inaccessible to local people. Through the agriculture ministry, new types of fences were developed and installed that allowed the ivy to grow waist high, permitting access by local people. The program was facilitated by a social marketing campaign and by involvement of agriculture officials with the local people. I think a program like that should be looked at as an example of one way to do it. The program is supervised by Mahidol University, is implemented in northeast Thailand, and supported by US AID.

Timothy Morck: Dr. Underwood?

Barbara Underwood: I would just like to make another comment on this. I think we need to keep in mind in relation to these programs that it is not only just producing these appropriate sources of vitamin A and other nutrients at the home level that is important. It also requires an educational program to make sure that these nutrients get into the diets of the children of those families who are the vulnerable groups that need vitamin A. In some of these areas, these appropriate foods are available, but they are not being properly used for child feeding. You have to take that additional step and mount an educational effort to address the food habits and patterns of child feeding in these areas as well.

Norge Jerome: In that context, if I may add, that is where the ministry of education comes in. Its interventions helped to make the ivy gourd an integral part of food habits.

Timothy Morck: Dr. Horwitz?

Abraham Horwitz: I feel as if I am speaking for Tshire Maribe who was unable to participate in this discussion. I remember that she was insistent on the role of adequate information and the best available data to enlist the support of all sectors. Frankly, I doubt that ministries of agriculture, if not properly informed, would be aware of the devastating effects of vitamin A deficiency. I believe that it is the role of ministries of health to be actively involved. The need for a highly sophisticated data management process may be secondary. I think there is a need, however, for the ministries of health to keep all the other ministries informed through planning and by making the data available.

Timothy Morck: Clearly, Dr. Monckeberg's description of the success of his program began with the element of the integration of the health system.

Fernando Monckeberg: That is correct.

Timothy Morck: Do you think that it is always going to be the case, that nutrition programs have to begin with health and from there share information with agriculture, the planners, and the economists?

Fernando Monckeberg: In my experience, I think this happens more in underdeveloped countries, that have a high percentage of the population that is marginalized from the economic and social structures of the society. The trouble is how to reach those people.

You have to develop a program, and the first problem is to find out where these people are, how many there are, and how to reach them. I think that the first way to reach them is through health. The best way would be to develop an adequate national health infrastructure. Through this infrastructure, you can reach them. This has been more or less our own experience.

Shubh Kumar: I would like to address the issue of the extent to which health ministries influence the economists, the planners, and the program developers. One thing I would point out would be the cost of this malnutrition, and I don't think we have addressed that enough. There was some work on this in the Asian context. In many areas, however, malnutrition, poverty, and poor health have not been seen as problems. I think we are facing up to that, and I think it is facing us much more directly. I do not think it is being addressed sufficiently.

In this context I should like to make a side comment on the work concerning human energy and its adaptation. It has been said that the term, adaptation, should not be used for other kinds of adjustments that are made. I think adaptation is a very positive thing and I think as long as adaptation is a good thing, there is no problem.

Judith McGuire: I would like to bring up another dimension of the issue: the role of agricultural research and of the international agricultural research centers in expanding health and nutrition. I myself have been struggling to define the most appropriate role for agricultural research in this. I know, maybe twenty-five years ago, agricultural researchers were looking into the protein aspects of growing corn.

I am wondering if there is a new impetus within agricultural research to think about either the qualitative aspects of the crops, how to increase consumption, and how to bring nutrient content and consumer issues into agricultural research, as opposed to production issues only.

Robert Chandler: In the case of rice, which feeds half of the world's population, when we started some thirty years ago, we thought that one of the things that we wanted to do was to increase the protein content of rice. As you know, the lysine content is high compared to other cereal grains. We did put a lot of effort into this and we found out there was a negative correlation between yield and protein content. When one went down, one went up, and vice versa. We were never able to get any varieties with more than 10 percent protein of dry weight. Normally, it was 7.5 to 8 percent, depending on what we could maintain, and depending on whether we got good yields.

As far as other aspects of nutrition in rice, it has been known for a long time that if you eat unpolished rice, you get along better than eating polished rice. But there are some real problems eating unpolished rice. One is that the oil content of the bran is so high that, under tropical conditions, if you mill it and let it sit as unpolished rice, then you get rancidness. It spoils in the tropical climate. Also, the people in the tropics have complained of digestive disturbances when they eat unpolished rice. They get some diarrhea. But we are talking about quality. You know about maize and there has been research done about that. We had problems with yield and climate, but then the research came in.

Still, the big problem is food security itself and the production of food in relation to the increasing world population. I feel certain that the greatest threat to the well-being of the world and mankind is the continuing high population growth rate. We develop all sorts of food production programs, but we haven't been able to keep up worldwide and we won't be able to keep up for long with the population growth.

For cereal grains, particularly rice and wheat, in the past twenty-five or thirty years, production has doubled. That has been good, yet the population has tripled. In Asia, production more than kept up with the population growth up until 1985 or

142

1986, somewhere along in there, and then the population numbers went beyond the grain production numbers.

Another thing which is disturbing to me is the fact that the planting areas devoted to the cereal grains have leveled off and, in some places, have even decreased. We did note an increase in the area devoted to rice in Asia around 1977, but it was low for that. In Africa, per capita food production has been going down since about 1967. The fact is that an increase in grain supply depends on an increase in yield rather than an increase in area for production. To me, this is a very serious problem.

Timothy Morck: I am not sure that you addressed Judith McGuire's comment about the role of these international agricultural research institutes in relation to nutrition.

Robert Chandler: I was trying to give the example of rice at an international research center. I think that the role of the international center is a very important one and has to do with both the quality and quantity of food, but within limits. To the extent that research can find ways of developing or creating varieties that are more nutritious, that is to the good. Emphasis also has to be given to the importance of a balanced diet. To me, the whole thing comes down to education.

We see countries where there has been progress, where there has been increasing production, decreasing poverty, and improved family planning programs. These have been the same countries where there is a high level of education.

On the other hand, there are countries with as few as 10 percent of the population being literate. In these situations it is very difficult to get health and nutrition programs going, whether it is growing more vegetables, or a balanced diet, or whatever.

As you know, I was director of the Asian Vegetable Research and Development Center in Taiwan, and we made the statement many times that vegetables are the greatest source of natural proteins, minerals, and vitamins. They are very important, and I think everybody realizes the need for more vegetables in the diet, that is, fruits and vegetables.

If the international agricultural research centers can play this role as they try to increase production, productivity, and yield, I think it would be beneficial. However, I think we have improved the food quality of a variety of cereal grains as much as probably can be done. As far as that goes, I think we have reached a plateau in this regard.

Timothy Morck: Dr. Greaves, do you have a comment?

Peter Greaves: First of all, picking up on Judith's question about the kind of work that international research institutes should be doing. It seems to me that an important question in the context of a particular country has to do with the employment situation in and the resources that are available to agriculture. What kind of agriculture are we trying to promote?

I have in mind a study that came from the National Academy of Sciences, the National Research Council, entitled "Alternative Agriculture." It is an extraordinarily interesting document. The *New York Times* devoted part of a front page to it. What it said was that after several years of study and after looking at several areas in the United States, the direction that agricultural production has been going for the past several years is the wrong one. It was going in a direction that was extremely demanding of resources, that was characterized by the excessive use of pesticides and fertilizers, and that was polluting the environment. A big question is whether one should be looking at agriculture in a very different way.

This study impressed me because it so happened around that time, I had been visiting Burma. At breakfast at the hotel in Rangoon, there was a newspaper article about a debate the day before in the Burmese parliament arguing that farmers would have to use many more pesticides and much more fertilizer. I wondered how long it would take for new thinking in one part of the world to penetrate to another part of the world. This is a very serious thing. Maybe one should be thinking in terms of systems of agriculture, which employ lots of people, rather than a few.

In the United States, the kind of agriculture that exists is agriculture that is intensive in all sorts of inputs, particularly capital inputs, but not in terms of people. But in much of the third world, it should be the other way around because so many people need employment. Maybe there should be the sort of agriculture that makes the maximum use of local resources, of composting and that sort of thing, and with a minimum reliance on pesticides and fertilizers because they are expensive, difficult to use, and potentially harmful to the environment. That is my first comment.

My second comment relates to a remark of Dr. Chandler's, which was extremely interesting, about the experience with rice and the kind of qualities that were built in. To me, it illustrates the importance of having a sound understanding of what the problems are. It is easy to look back with hindsight, of course. I am not being critical at all of the decisions that were made. It seems that in this kind of situation, one might be seeking the maximum yield because more food was needed, even if that jeopardized an increase in the protein content. Maybe that is not a wise payoff.

I am reminded of one of the factors that led to the end of World War I. The conventional wisdom at the time in Germany was that soldiers needed lots of meat. They needed it to fight. So, for years the agricultural policy of Germany was geared to provide meat to soldiers. Consequently, there wasn't too much food for the people and there was a very serious food shortage, which hastened the end of the war. I'm reminded of the phrase, "do you want beef for some or bread for all?" And they chose beef for some and, consequently, there wasn't enough bread for all.

The third comment comes back to Miss Maribe's paper. She highlights the link between malnutrition and the problem of food access, which continues to be a major obstacle. The only point I want to make is that in my view we must be careful to distinguish the problems of food production and of access to food. Both factors can lead to malnutrition. However, though a household may have access to food, children may not consume it, or they may be suffering from infection that affects their thyroid and their ability to utilize the food they do consume. So, as I tried to say yesterday, food production, food access, and health care are all necessary. None is sufficient alone; all are important.

Timothy Morck: I would like to give Dr. Chandler an opportunity to respond to that, and then Dr. Yeung has a comment.

Robert Chandler: Let me respond to your comment about composting and fertilizer use. The former is a sound practice, but it may not be able to maintain a particularly high yield. For example, China was the greatest recirculator of organic matter in the world, without any question. When I was in China in 1977, however, they were building thirteen chemical fertilizer plants in the country because they could not get their rice to grow without chemical fertilizers as well as organic. This is one of the problems; there are limits to organic fertilizer because you can't convert all organic matter. Things are taken out, things are eaten, things are thrown away, and you waste a great deal, and so forth. Probably, we cannot feed the world in the long run without using chemical fertilizer. I think that is true.

We also can't feed the world in the long run without much more use of irrigation water than is the case at the present time. There is no question about that. The Niger River in West Africa, in Guinea, is in an area with almost 200 inches of rainfall a year. Yet if you go into the hinterland hundreds of miles, you find that very little of that water is used in growing food. They are trying to use the Senegal River now. This is a problem throughout Africa.

I do feel that food quality is important and the increasing population is a problem and, of course, people need jobs. I am very much concerned about India and China because they are having rather difficult times with the population problem there. The population problem is acute. India always has had a well-educated class of people, but it also has a low literacy rate among the population as a whole. That shows the problems that they have there. There was an article in the paper in the past few weeks that the government was attempting to get the lower class more jobs in government and the people who already have jobs are rioting. Overpopulation is a real problem, the basic problem.

So, this is a very serious thing that we face. Until there is a will on the part of governments and a will on the part of foreign assistance agencies in the United States of America and elsewhere to mount massive family planning programs, I don't know how we are going to solve these problems.

Timothy Morck: Dr. Yeung?

David Yeung: I just wanted to respond to Peter Greaves's first comment and respond to the part about China using organic fertilizers. There are a lot of chemical fertilizers being used in China and it is scary. Of course, there is more of a demand for more food in China and India, but it has always been an open policy. The families in China are growing more food and see an advantage in selling it, so consequently they are looking for a greater yield. And that's when they go into the chemical fertilizers.

In terms of composting, in the African Sahel, where I spent a little time, we taught some of the local people how to compost, how to have home gardens, and it worked on a small space. But the basic problem is still water. We still need water in the desert for the crops. You have to compete for the water with the need of people to drink, and water is given to the animals. None is left for farming.

Going back to the question of iron deficiency and vitamin A deficiency, there is iron deficiency prevalent worldwide. If you go back a few years, iron deficiency was even more prevalent, but it has been brought under control, particularly in the industrialized countries. In some Third World countries, particularly in China, they have basically eradicated iron deficiency, except, of course, in the more remote areas. For some reason, we have not been entirely successful because it is still prevalent in the world, including North America.

Timothy Morck: Did you say that iron deficiency has been eradicated in China?

David Yeung: I meant iodine deficiency.

Timothy Morck: Thank you. I thought there wasn't enough delineation there. So, iodine deficiency has been eliminated?

David Yeung: In the more remote areas, it is still there. In the areas where there is some concentration, it has been minimized. I wonder why it is the case that we have been readily successful with iodine, but not as successful when it comes to iron. That has been bothering me quite a bit. For instance, in North America, we have been able to control, minimize, or even eradicate vitamin deficiencies, but not iron deficiency.

Timothy Morck: Dr. Kahn, that's a good lead-in.

Samuel Kahn: I'm going to go back to what Judith McGuire said a little while ago about agriculture research centers. I wonder what is the involvement with nutrition at these centers. I know they do agricultural research. I know in past years there have been elaborate activities with some nutrition groups, but some of these programs at the agricultural research centers have not been continued.

I was wondering if any of the agricultural research centers have a nutritional component, whether directly in their center or in collaboration with other nutrition-related institutes. I have a feeling that there is not strong collaboration. Maybe this is something that should be looked at in terms of strengthening the relationship, in terms of having a nutrition input in the research and in the products that come out of the centers. True, they have improved genetic material for other things besides protein that are important in certain foods. Also, it may make other agriculture researchers more aware that nutrition should be a concern of people who do research in agriculture and not just quantity, but the quality factor as well.

Changing direction, I think that iron deficiency is a problem that is difficult to address because you have in food, especially in vegetables, cereals, and legumes, some components that inhibit iron absorption. It is not that easy to introduce an iron component into a food. Also, when you think of iodine and iron, the amount of iodine you have to put into something is minuscule compared to the quantities of iron. You are talking micrograms versus milligrams in terms of putting supplements into food. You also have a problem of some reaction because iron is so interactive.

It is much more difficult to deal with iron because it is something humans need on a daily basis and the absorption of iron is very well controlled by the body. It stores it away. It does not take it up all at once like vitamin A. It only takes up so much. As I say, it is much more difficult to develop programs that will address iron deficiency because it is more difficult in terms of treatment and the amounts that are needed.

Timothy Morck: Dr. Horwitz had a question.

Abraham Horwitz: I think that Dr. Kahn said it much better, as usual. I would like to address the comment about the role of agricultural research centers in nutrition. The Advisory Group on Nutrition has tried to enlist the agricultural centers to do research in improving foods, but we have not got very far.

It brings to mind a presentation last year by Dr. Jerome on research on food varieties that are not expensive to produce, and I think that line of research is very valuable. But some of these issues are so complex from the research point of view that there may be the feeling that these concerns are not appealing. Yet we should persist.

Timothy Morck: Dr. Underwood has a question and then Dr. Jerome.

Barbara Underwood: I have a quick comment because I think this issue that we are addressing right now is very important. That is, the role of the international agricultural research centers. I am thinking particularly of the vegetable research center that you helped start, Dr. Chandler. In those early days, I had an opportunity to come and visit that center.

I recall at that time there was a recognition of the importance of nutrition and that a person be brought right on board—one of the reasons I was there is because they were trying to interview me to go there and be a part of that center. I had other commitments, but someone was brought in with a background in nutrition. I recall at that time that I had a concern about one of the products that was being promoted for Asia, the yam, the sweet potato.

Robert Chandler: Well, the sweet potato and the yam are two different things.

Barbara Underwood: I know, but the yam is primarily the one that was being promoted. The reason I bring it up is this. There were some choices, some trade-offs at that time, regarding the varieties. One was a much lighter kind of variety that seemed to have more yield than some of the darker orange varieties. It was a trade-off. Which do you go for? Also, the lighter variety in certain parts of that area was more acceptable to the population.

At the time, I think the consideration was one of yield and of the greater consumer preference for the lighter variety, as the critical factors for deciding what

147

to promote. But there were a number of countries in the area that had vitamin A deficiency and that did not consume very much of that yam, yet here was a chance of introducing a new healthful product into some of those countries.

We know now, for example, from some of the work that Dr. Rahmathullah is doing, to try to get to a group of children who have far more than clinical signs of vitamin A deficiency and that the vitamin loss is affecting the much larger population of children and their very chances of survival.

The reason I bring it up in relation to the international agriculture research centers is the matter of awareness. The awareness of what the magnitude of the problems are and of the economic and the human costs. So, I think we are entering into a new age when there is even more of a need to have people in nutrition involved in the international centers to bring out these issues, to keep the researchers up to date as to what are the human costs that need to be taken into consideration in deciding the directions to go and the crops, even varieties within crops, that are being promoted.

Norge Jerome: Basically, we are talking about both the quantity and the quality of the diet. Someone mentioned that the issue is food, and by producing an adequate supply of quality food, we really ought to be achieving the goals of reducing malnutrition and upgrading the nutritional well-being of people. I want it to be stated as clearly as possible that what has occurred in the past—the varieties versus protein debate—detracts from the goal at hand, which is to produce an adequate supply of food to individuals who must be adequately fed.

Let me move away from agriculture to other sectors. I was impressed by the paper that was presented yesterday by Miss Maribe, examining where nutrition is located in the various ministries. I was excited about it because my own office has just embarked on a search for that. Because our goal is multisectoral, we thought it was absolutely necessary to find out which ministries have a nutrition component, in the various countries. I think that is very important for implementation purposes, that we know which one does what, and, therefore, we can develop an appropriate implementation plan that engages each one of these various ministries.

I would also like some of you who work in various countries to elaborate a little bit more. Your responses were very brief yesterday on the topic of coordination and implementation. I think that is a very important topic. Do you mind elaborating on this some more because I think it is very important.

Abraham Horwitz: I think it is very difficult not to coordinate and implement. I think there are three things we have to consider. Not only for coordination and implementation, but also the elaboration, the detailed development of the program, that we want to be implemented.

My point of view is that not only does the program have to be implemented, but if you are to set down the details of the program, somewhere in the process of elaboration, you have to get in contact with those people who are going to implement it. If you get people involved in the whole problem in this way, they feel that it is their own problem. I don't believe it is easy to separate elaboration, coordination, and implementation.

Neil Kotler: Could I just ask you, elaboration means what, the definition of the problem? The measurement of the problem?

Abraham Horwitz: The ability to analyze a problem and to intervene and determine what has to be done. That is elaboration.

Norge Jerome: It also means maintenance of performance standards, once you have a program in place.

Robert Chandler: I am not an expert in nutrition, as you well know, but I do know that with the cereal grains, for example, wheat, maize, rice and sorghum, that you cannot do very much beyond trying to raise the protein content. I do not think there are many other things that you can do that I know about in increasing the nutritional quality of the product. We have seen that one of the real problems in malnutrition is the amount of carbohydrates that you take in as well as protein. Poverty is the great scourge in less developed countries. Economically speaking, the countries that have shown economic development have also demonstrated agricultural productivity and increasing income. So, we do what we can to provide more food and more income so that people can live better.

Now, when it comes to the vegetable center in Taiwan, one of the primary considerations was to increase the nutritional value of these crops and also to achieve crop tolerance to warm temperatures, characteristic of the tropics. These are the areas in the world where much of the poverty and much of the malnutrition in the world is concentrated. Take the example of Chinese cabbage. In Taiwan, the cabbage could grow only in the winter months, but we couldn't get a tolerance in the summertime. Limits on the size of the soybean crop is another example. At certain times of the year, it depended on the rainfall.

I would just like to say that, while I think nutrition is very important, I do not see what these research centers can do when they are working with the cereal grains. I do not know what the possibility is of increasing the nutritional value of cassava, for example, which, of course, is grown a great deal in Latin America and in Africa. We have seen a great deal of malnutrition in poor, young children who were brought up on cassava. In Colombia under a Rockefeller Foundation program, we saw that the yam, the true yam, not the sweet potato, is not a good source of vitamins and minerals. It is a source of carbohydrates, but it is low in protein. We have no problems with the root crops.

By all means, we need home gardens, places where you can grow crops, even up on the roofs of houses in urban areas. People can produce their vegetables there. However, in many cases the people are so poor that they sell their crops rather than eat them, and that is another problem. One of the papers yesterday pointed out that the most severe problems were in the rural areas, not the urban. You keep finding in lesser developed countries that the most severe poverty is in the rural areas, not in the urban.

Timothy Morck: Dr. McGuire?

Judith McGuire: I am afraid that incorporating nutrition into agricultural research requires a total rethinking of what we are calling agricultural research. I think the research into the genetics of the crops is going to contribute very little, although I can think of one problem that it might answer. That is trying to breed a low phytate, low tannin grain which might have a less inhibitory effect on iron absorption.

I think we really have to think about production systems and income differentiation and the processing and handling of grain in agriculture. It is not just a matter of growing a high-yielding crop, as much as growing a mix of crops that meets a number of needs, including nutrient needs.

Also important are the human energy requirements to grow it, as well as the human time requirements. Gender is a factor. Is it the women's time, is it the men's time? I think in Africa we really need to think about something to grow during the *hungry season*, the period preceding harvest time when food stores are low, because in a lot of these countries, the nutrition problem is most acute in the hungry season. Is there something we can do about the very low level of water? The water harvesting idea, somehow growing crops in the off-season, should be explored. I know in Kenya, for instance, there has been a transition from sorghum to maize. This is the worst thing you can do in terms of vulnerability to drought. They now have a food security problem that they didn't have before the transition.

We need to think about the cooking qualities of the foods that we are growing. You mentioned the problem of milled rice versus unmilled rice. One of the biggest differences is that unmilled rice requires twice the cooking time. Where we have a firewood problem and where we also have women's time constraints, the cooking time for grains may be a key determinant of nutrition, irrespective of the nutritional quality of a specific grain, or a specific commodity that agricultural research is focusing on.

Finally, we nutritionists tend to put a lot of blame on agricultural researchers when, in reality, we often do not know what to do. I am hard-pressed to think about what I would do if I were an agricultural researcher. How can I help them to do a better job of addressing nutrition? I am a little skeptical that we have the answers.

Timothy Morck: We can state the problems, but the answers are harder to come by. Dr. Greaves has a comment and then Dr. Kahn.

Peter Greaves: The point I want to make is that if an agricultural research institute is developing something new, it is equally challenging to try to distribute it and get it consumed. Our feeling is that many of these institutes conceive their role primarily on the production side, and that is it. They are not too concerned about extension work. Research institutes ought to be concerned to follow through from production to actual consumption, taking into account the properties of a food, consumption, and so forth. Dr. Underwood made the point earlier that if the food is not consumed, it is not any good.

150

We have talked about the Asian Vegetable Institute that Dr. Chandler was associated with. There is an institute in West Africa, and I have forgotten the name of it, which has done a lot of work on cassava. It produced a variety that has many positive features about it; not particularly nutritional ones, but features that make it more drought resistant and resistant to diseases. At one point, UNICEF had discussions with this institute on ways to help promote this variety, moving from the research confines to actual use. To be honest, it was a very frustrating experience. It was extremely hard to get a response to this, apart from one or two individuals. It seems to be a critically important point that one must follow through and be concerned with the communications aspect and make sure that there are people on the staff who understand the implications for nutrition and health. There is little good if you cannot communicate it.

Samuel Kahn: I would like to follow up on something that Peter Greaves said, and that is, where do we start? In discussions I have had with colleagues covering agriculture, I have a sense that for agriculturalists their end person is the farmer. In nutrition, the end person is the consumer, the person who eats the food. I think this is a gap and this is why we may approach things and see things differently. I think we have to bring that together and encourage the people in agriculture to go further beyond where their products are going to go. It is not just an increase in production for the farmer, but also increasing the quality of the products for the consumer. That should be the measure of success.

With reference to the products that come out of agricultural research centers, yes, they have improved amino acid profiles of certain cereals. We found some years ago that when you start to analyze the genetic components of the cereal, if you factor in chemical components, improvement may be seen in different compartments of that product. When you feed it to an individual, and we were dealing with young children who respond well to good nutrition and this was our measuring stick, we found, however, that many of the improved products had poor digestibility because the amino acid improvements were in the components that were not digested well.

So, we had products that looked very good on paper, from the chemical analysis stand point and the agricultural reports, but they were poor performers in terms of nutritional merit. My conclusion is that many of these products that look good, are resistant to pests, have good chemical profiles, need, in addition, nutrition testing at the research centers. The research centers really do not go far enough.

Timothy Morck: Neil Kotler, a comment?

Neil Kotler: If I may, I would like to engage Dr. Liu and Dr. Rahmathullah, and Dr. Monckeberg around the following issue. To play devil's advocate, it has been said that Chile has been a very successful country in terms of nutrition, education, and behavior change. If we compare Chile to India and China, I would submit that Chile is very different and I wonder how generalizable the Chilean experience is. It is different in at least two ways. Unless I am ignorant of this because I have not been to Chile, ethnically, and racially, and culturally, it is rather homogeneous, whereas China and India are very heterogenous. Secondly, Chile has twelve million people. China has over one billion, and India, nearly one billion.

Thirty years ago when I was in college, Sweden was viewed as an exemplary success story, combining socialism and capitalism. Even then, I remember Sweden was an exceptional case. It was homogeneous and rather small. How can you generalize that experience to India and China? How do you develop nutrition and health programs in large countries with culturally diverse, disparate, different peoples? How do you communicate, distinctively, with these different subcultures?

Liu Dong-sheng: I think there have been changes in China. Of course, China is different politically from your country, I don't know how to say it, because my work lies in nutritional research. There are problems encountered. My work does not always provide good results, good effects for the children. That is the problem.

Now, our children have iron deficiency and calcium deficiency, these two deficiencies. If we can do some work on these problems, we can do good for the children. We have established a coordination committee that works with women and children, and directly with the state council. Through this committee, different agencies such as the ministry of health, can coordinate with people and organizations and they can work together. So, I think this committee will work for change. We have established the committee just in this past year.

Neil Kotler: I suppose I am asking you because China has so many different kinds of people, languages, racial and cultural backgrounds. You are saying that programs are reaching people, irrespective of cultural differences? It's just a matter of finding ways to have effective programs to reach the target, the children?

David Yeung, I don't know if you can help us out here. You have much experience in China. Any problems in undertaking communications and behavioral interventions with regard to so many disparate peoples?

David Yeung: Yesterday, somebody used the terms, political cost, political benefit. I think that is very important. That is extremely important in China. In recent history, there has been a fair amount of emphasis on improving the health and income of minorities in China. For instance, the one family, one child policy is basically for the Han people, the Chinese people in the urban areas. Whereas, if you are in a minority group, you may be able to have more than one child.

That is extremely important to China because the minorities live in the border areas. They provide the stability that is important to China, between China itself and the bordering countries. You have to have a stable population that will be loyal to the country. In terms of that equation, the political benefit is extremely important in China. They are willing to spend more time and more money to promote the health of these minorities.

That goes back to what I said before in terms of iron and iodine. It is related to that as well, possibly because of the fact that iodine is easily recognized, whereas iron deficiency is not. So, consequently, if you can minimize the problem of iodine deficiency, you seem to be doing a good thing. Whereas even though you are improving the iron problem, it is not seen that easily. That is another equation that is related to politics.

V. Rahmathullah: In India, actually the issue of diverse cultures is sorted out by the different states. The states decide on how to develope distinctive education programs. They deal directly with the ethnic groups in advocating a nutrition program. We cannot have a generalized nutrition program for the whole country. We have to do it state by state.

Timothy Morck: Dr. Monckeberg, would you like to conclude this particular line of discussion?

Fernando Monckeberg: It would be impossible for me to discuss how other programs in other countries are run. In other countries, the degree of development may be different, and also the income per capita may be very different. You start from different points and these differences are important to consider. The amount of the total population is much simpler when you have a population of twelve million rather than one billion.

Now, you have to consider the concentration, or density, of the people. You have to consider the percentage of rural population versus the percentage of urban population, and where they are located. Many people think that Chile is a very long and narrow country. In one sense, it is true. Yet only 19 percent or so of the population lives in the rural parts of the country. Because the country is not wide, it is much easier to work with the population because it is concentrated. Approximately 80 percent of the Chilean population is urban. There are other differences too. This situation is completely different from situations in other countries.

My point is that it is important to recognize and learn from the successful cases, to analyze their approaches and technology. On the other hand, every country has to study its own reality. This has to be studied from a particular point of view. I think it is important to have adequate numbers of people preparing a diagnostic study of possible health and nutrition intervention. That involves doing the basic research and applying the research in the operations phase. I think it is important to analyze the circumstances in each country in developing a program and to organize all groups in order to justify support for the intervention. We have heard a lot about specific nutrient deficiencies, such as iron, or vitamin A, or iodine. In my point of view, you have to study each of them and target a program to each particular disorder.

Some of these nutrition problems affect mainly children below six years of age. Now, you can develop a program where you can bring all these things together and target them to young children. You can use this as a mechanism to solve the nutrient deficiency. If you organize an effective and targeted program, you can reduce costs. However, this kind of thing has to be analyzed in each particular country. You cannot take one program and put it in another country.

Even in Latin America, for example, in Peru, there are tremendous problems that arise from the rural character of the country. A large percentage of the people do not speak Spanish. So, there are different problems to confront in each country.

Judith McGuire: I think when we look at successful cases in large countries like Brazil and Mexico, as well as in China and India, a pattern emerges. I think in those countries where programs have worked, you find a strong central leadership in nutrition, for example INCA in Brazil or the National Institute of Nutrition in India. Furthermore, there also is a pattern of strong decentralization. One finds organizations that perform well, and this has something to do with literacy and education. This observation echoes a point Dr. Chandler was making. There certainly is motivation in evidence. In the cases where you do have this decentralization, you also might find areas of the country which are underdeveloped, such as is the case in northeast Brazil or in Nigeria.

I think you need a combination of localized control, localized motivation, as well as strong central leadership on the part of some group at the center that can, in fact, help to reduce or minimize the inequities that exist among regions. In northeast Brazil, São Paulo is doing an excellent job. They have got a lot of resources and they do not need the central leadership to do it. Even in the United States, one finds the south is much poorer than the northeast—though that is changing with the changes in the economy. You have to have a nutrition goal embedded in the centralized system and at the same time there has to be decentralized administration. I think that China is an interesting example, a case where central control has worked to eliminate famine, but this has left a number of inequities among regions in terms of overall well-being. It is not easy to say that Chile is or is not a model for someone else. On the other hand, it is useful to look at specific aspects of the Chilean experience, which has worked successfully.

Timothy Morck: This, I think, is a good point to lead into a comment I made earlier. I want to ask Dr. Roberto to look at the communication aspect of nutrition programs. Would you like to comment?

Eduardo Roberto: I guess you can look at the issue of what works and does not work in different cultures and view it from the standpoint of the people who are responsible for the programs, or else from the standpoint of the consumers of a program's services. You have to understand the simple things even in the most complex situations.

One of the things that I have learned from those who implement social programs is that when you talk about different cultures, different people, those differences count only to the extent that they are causally linked. Those differences might reflect differences in needs and behavior. In other words, what we have seen in Chile may not be something that we want to do in China or in India. However, if there are different groups who have the same need for the same program in the same period, you would have to treat them the same, even if they have different cultures.

I think what I have learned from implementers in this regard is that we must differentiate between the result of what we have done and the process of doing it. I think the problem was raised by Dr. Monckeberg when he said that you need to be looking at how to make things effective, and the first order of business is to understand the target group that a program seeks to reach. Research is a key factor for success.

In other words, you do not want to use the model of Chile simply in terms of replicating the results. You want to use the experience of Chile as a process, a process of taking a first step, a second step, and so on. And the first step is to understand the people whom you want to help. I think that is simply the case. Whenever I examine a program, the very first thing I have to understand is who is the target group, the beneficiary group, what is being done now to help those people, and what problems are we trying to resolve.

Let me comment on the other point that was raised about coordination and elaboration. How do you look at the coordination of ministries, at intergovernmental relationships, from the standpoint of social marketing? I made the comment yesterday that you can think of those groups as a target segment, but whose behavior do you want to change? Yesterday, in fact, Dr. Monckeberg mentioned this point in terms of attempting to influence the various presidential candidates in Chile, to win their support for nutrition and health programs. He analyzed their needs to have political power, to be visible, and to be reelected, and he designed a product or a communication around these needs. He says to each one, I want to give you the tools to get that power. To that extent, each presidential candidate is a market segment of one person. Let me draw from that. You do have a target. You do have a product. You are promoting and persuading. You are promoting an adoption to one and the same person, in this case a presidential candidate.

Of course, it is a different matter when you talk about program sustainability and about program coordination. What about the continuing relationship of one group with another, one ministry with another? What I have found is that implementation is almost an abstraction, something that does not exist in pure form. It's a convenient expectation. In reality, implementers plan, they organize, they promote and negotiate, they improvise, and they try to make adjustments. When you give something to an implementer, that individual will go through a planning and a re-planning cycle.

The question has to do with linkages, with coordination among government agencies, in order to produce an efficient program. In the Philippines a program may be in the hands of an agency, but this agency does not have the facilities for doing the work. Another ministry may be in charge. What you need is to relate to the other agencies, to persuade them that it is for their own good to cooperate. An implementer may not have the authority, but he or she does have the responsibility to implement an efficient program. For instance, consider the example of our family planning program. One particular agency may not have the authority or the facilities to get it done.

This is a perfect setting for doing social marketing. There are three items to consider. You want a performance out of the program, but performance is both a process and a skill. The process is clear. You have to map out where and what role each of the different government agencies will have to play. But the important part is still the skilled manager.

For the program implementer, it often is difficult to relate to a particular government agency, or a ministry. It is difficult because you cannot just stand before a building and say, "I want to relate to you." But you can plan that on Monday morning you will speak to Mr. X or Ms. Y at the ministry. You have to determine, who is there to speak to? When one is talking about people in a government agency, there are two kinds of things that one has to look for. Who is going to be the program champion at a particular ministry? Who sincerely believes that what you are doing is beneficial and is to the benefit of his or her own agency? You sell not only your point of view, but you also have to let him know how it would benefit him.

Once you have a product champion, you have to ascertain his status. Does this champion have a benevolent benefactor? How does he stand with the head of the agency? I think it is extremely important to have support to do the job, and to do the job, you must have the coordination. It is important to have that. So, the important thing is trying to determine who is going to be the product champion. But I learned from Dr. Monckeberg that the way to get there is to make sure that the successive political leaders are people whom you know.

Neil Kotler: If you would indulge me one more minute. There are two sides to the equation of social marketing. Social marketing is an exchange relationship. We have been focusing on the target group, the consumer, the client. How about the provider, namely the health workers, the bureaucrats, the authorities at the top? How do you motivate the provider side in implementing an effective intervention? Health and nutrition programs are among the most labor-intensive operations in the world, having all kinds of intricate contact situations, and relying heavily on providers of services. If I have any reservation about social marketing, it has to do with the provider side of the marketing equation. How do you motivate the providers of these services?

Eduardo Roberto: Let me answer that. If you look at an interagency relationship, those are your providers. Once you look at them from the social marketing standpoint, you are looking at them as if they are your consumers, your clients. They have needs of their own. So, when I am looking for the product champion, I am trying to shortcut the process of having to do a lot of research with regard to the levels of power and influence. I need to get the job done now. I want to find somebody whose motivations coincide with what I need done in implementing a program. Suppose I do not find one? Then I do the research, basically intelligence research. I go around and I find out who are the people with influence, and what their needs are. Let me illustrate this idea.

I got into trouble once in the Philippines because, as predicted, the church organizations were going to go against the program I was working on. My assignment was to promote a national program for contraception. My first assignment was getting large numbers of people to make use of condoms. I listed all of the influence groups that would be potentially affected by the program. The first was a Catholic group called Couples for Christ. Another one was Christian Family Living. I had to find out who would be the program critics. What I did was to find out who are the people who have a say in these organizations. I had all of the people listed.

When the project was launched, a Catholic women's group had many people criticizing the program. I had to find a way to neutralize the critics. My boss said that I was in trouble, but I expected that. He asked me what I intended to do about it. I told him to give me seventy-two hours to resolve it and, if I don't resolve it, I'll resign. I went through my lists and I found out who was in charge. I found out it was a woman who was a court officer, a judge. I knew I had to talk to her and I had to sell her on the program. I had to find out what her needs were. My objective at that time was to find out everything about her.

I first asked if I could talk to her and try to flush out the problem. She did not agree. Then I discovered the high school boyfriend of the judge was a friend of mine. So, I went up to him and said that he owed me a favor, and that I'm collecting now. I wanted him to get for me just a half an hour appointment with the judge. I simply wanted to find out from her what was wrong with my campaign. I thought it was pretty good. I got to meet her, and I found out the problem was a lack of communication. I got to talk to her, and she told me that I was promoting a program with only one birth control method. The Church had agreed, on the other hand, to a family planning program that allowed for use of many different methods. You are advertising your condoms, front page, every day, she said. That is only one method, so you are violating the agreement.

Let me sum up this experience. The judge said the condom advertisement was about a single birth control method, and it excluded others such as natural family planning. So, that was the nub of the issue, the lack of communication. I am happy to report we revised the advertising and communications, and won the support of the judge. It is the basic approach that is simple—namely, know your consumer, your target group. If it is going to be a provider, a government agency, or a powerful individual, treat the provider as the consumer.

Timothy Morck: Thank you. Did you have a brief comment, Dr. Greaves?

Peter Greaves: I am fascinated by the details of these stories. To me, an important thing to come out of this colloquium is a kind of process in helping to empower communities to do things themselves. I disagree, however, with your distinction between provider versus beneficiary. That is true for certain things such as immunization or providing birth control pills to women. But these problems are different from malnutrition problems, which have to do with basic survival. The time constraints on women and all that kind of thing leads me to conclude that successful programs ultimately depend on community action.

Miss Maribe's paper referred to community information systems. What can one do to help communities help themselves? Our language often fails us. Her paper frequently uses the term "food and nutrition service." This has a top-down connotation, that may be appropriate in some situations, but not in the more basic ones. I remember at a meeting several years go, a phrase was used, "delivery of integrated services." That's the wrong phrase. The real concern is to generate interrelated activity.

David Yeung: I just want to go back to what Dr. Roberto has mentioned about being a provider. In the case of a firm or an industry that is in partnership with other sectors in society, in the delivering or marketing of a service, I think we see examples where this can be looked at objectively. Industry support of ILSI is an example of how an industry can work to bring a service or product to the community.

We have done that very well in China, but there is a lot still to be done. The Heinz Institute in China is a facility for the support of scientists in China. We do that with the cooperation of scientists in China, of scientists in North America, and, in some cases, in Europe as well. The advantage is, that we have the resources of the company behind us and we can have access to the marketing know-how and the marketing network. I think that is extremely important. I wonder, Dr. Rahmathullah, as we talked about it yesterday, in the case of vitamin A in India and the problems that you are experiencing in terms of delivering the information and the goods that you have, whether you have considered working with the local food industry. Sometimes, it can be extremely useful because they have the marketing know-how and the network.

V. Rahmathullah: Actually, the food industry is not that active. The food industry produces food that is rather expensive and geared to the elite group. The poor people depend on the local markets and on the home gardens. So, a relationship with industry has little to offer. I do not think that the food industry linkage would be beneficial in our case.

David Yeung: I found in China that the Heinz Company has generated some competition in relation to the baby food industry. People are saying, why is there just one company to make all the financial gains? Why can't we do it ourselves? That has prompted local industry to come forward and say they can do it, too. Maybe we can challenge the local food industries to come out with some ideas and the local people would benefit.

Timothy Morck: Our time has run out, unfortunately, and I just have a couple of closing comments. This whole discussion has appropriately come back to the community level. We started out there and we have gone into far-reaching issues of agricultural research institutes, regional institutes, industry, and government structures, and yet we have come back to the community level at the close. We firmly believe, I think collectively in this room, that the sustainable programs are those that are built upon community action.

One comment about what Dr. Roberto was saying about marketing to the providers. I think the point that made that effective in Dr. Monckeberg's situation, making the message a tool for the politicians, was based on the fact that consumers, the public in general, already had recognized the nutrition program as something they would be willing to vote for. So, I don't think it would have been effective in the absence of community support for the need for good nutrition. That was what gave the politicians the power to do that.

In the various programs that the Nutrition Foundation manages for the Office of Nutrition at US AID, there is a strong sense that community-level activity has to be promoted. It is appropriate, therefore, that our vitamin A conference in June will focus on community-based vitamin A programs, and this will be an opportunity to explore these avenues for approaching the vitamin A problem through different systems operating at the community level.

I heard a number of points today in talking about community programs that actually were examined in a workshop that Dr. Norge Jerome was instrumental in convening in 1989, the title of which was "Crucial Elements of Successful Community Nutrition Programs." On the back table, there are books with the proceedings of that conference, and I encourage you to review the materials.

One final comment. Communication is truly a theme that weaves through all of this, at every level: the idea of information being exchanged, not just through education, not just in giving out information, but making sure that it is received and embodied by those whom you are trying to convince or contact. This is so important that the International Nutrition Planners Forum has set for its 1991 meeting the topic of "Effective Communication for Behavioral Change." I am encouraged that some of the thinking that I have heard around this table can be incorporated into that program.

There is a need to look at the nutrition programs in a particular country, to look at their program leaders, and where their information is coming from to support their mission. The program mission, as we have seen, is two-fold, involving providers and consumers, and then linking both to people who are specialists in communications. I think that is really the kind of coordination and integration that is going to prove to be successful, and that we need to encourage.

On that note, I will close and thank each one of you for your active participation today. We have touched on many topics that we began to examine yesterday. We have gone beyond that and discovered other issues as well. We have had a very productive discussion. Each one of you, I thank very much.

APPENDIX A

Colloquium Program,
October 17, 1990

9:00 AM   Welcoming Remarks

Robert McC. Adams, Secretary, Smithsonian Institution
Alex Malaspina, President, International Life Sciences Institute-Nutrition Foundation

9:20 AM–12:30 PM   Morning Session: *Research Frontiers of Nutrition and Food Security*

V. Rahmathullah, Director, Child Development Unit, Aravind Children's Hospital, Madurai, India
"Effects of Frequent, Low-Dose Vitamin A Intake on Child Survival: Implications for Community-Based Programs"
Liu Dong-sheng, Professor of Nutrition, Chinese Academy of Preventive Medicine, Beijing, People's Republic of China
"Strategies to Combat Iron Deficiency Anemia in China"
Tshire Olivia Maribe, Chief Nutritionist, Ministry of Health, Gaborone, Republic of Botswana
"Household-Level Food and Nutrition Security in the East, Central and Southern Africa Region"
Discussants:
J. Peter Greaves, Senior Adviser (Micronutrients), Programme Division, United Nations Children's Fund (UNICEF), New York, New York

Judith S. McGuire, Nutritionist, Population, Health, and Nutrition Division, The
World Bank, Washington, D.C.
Session Chair:
Barbara A. Underwood, Assistant Director for International Program Activities,
National Eye Institute, National Institutes of Health, Bethesda, Maryland

12:30 PM   Luncheon

2:00 PM–4:45 PM   Afternoon Session: *Strategies for Nutrition and Food Security:
Perspectives on Policy, Programs, and Behavioral Intervention*

Fernando Monckeberg B., Director, Instituto de Nutrición y Tecnología de los
Alimentos, Universidad de Chile, Santiago, Chile
"Integrating National Food, Nutrition, and Health Policy: The Chilean Experience"
Eduardo L. Roberto, Coca-Cola Foundation Professor of International Marketing,
Asian Institute of Management, Manila, The Philippines
"Changing Health and Nutrition Behavior: A Social Marketing View"
Discussants:
Abraham Horwitz, Director Emeritus, Pan American Sanitary Bureau, Pan Ameri-
can Health Organization, Washington, D.C.
David L. Yeung, Corporate Nutrition Coordinator, H.J. Heinz Company of Canada
Ltd., North York, Ontario, Canada
Session Chair:
Norge W. Jerome, Director, Office of Nutrition, Bureau for Science and Technology,
U.S. Agency for International Development, Washington, D.C.

Colloquium Summation

Barbara A. Underwood, Assistant Director for International Program Activities,
National Eye Institute, National Institutes of Health, Bethesda, Maryland

6:30 PM   The World Food Prize Award Ceremony, Baird Auditorium, National
Museum of Natural History

John S. Niederhauser, World Food Prize Laureate, 1990, Acceptance Address

7:30 PM   Buffet Reception

APPENDIX B

Notes on Contributors

Robert F. Chandler, Jr.

Robert F. Chandler, Jr., founding director, International Rice Research Institute, the Philippines. Educated at the University of Maine and the University of Maryland (Ph.D., 1934). Held several posts at the Rockefeller Foundation: as associate director for agricultural sciences; assistant director, natural science and agriculture; soil scientist with the Mexican Agricultural Program. Directed the Asian Vegetable Research and Development Center in Taiwan. Served as dean of the College of Agriculture and as president of the University of New Hampshire. Professor of forest soils at Cornell University; state horticulturist at the Maine State Department of Agriculture. Author of *An Adventure in Applied Research: A History of the International Rice Research Institute* (1982); *Rice in the Tropics: A Guide to Development of National Programs* (1979); and *Forest Soils,* with Harold J. Lutz (1946), along with some sixty articles in professional and trade journals. Recipient, The World Food Prize (1988), U.S. Presidential End Hunger Award (1986), Special Award of the Republic of China (1975), International Agronomy Award (1972), Golden Heart of the Republic of the Philippines (1972), Star of Merit of the Republic of Indonesia (1972), Star of Distinction Award of the Government of Pakistan (1968), and Gold Medal of the Government of India (1966). Awarded eight honorary degrees from universities throughout the world. Born in Columbus, Ohio, 1907. Address: P. O. Box 852, Raymond, ME 04071.

J. Peter Greaves

J. Peter Greaves, senior adviser in the programme division (micronutrients), United Nations Children's Fund (UNICEF). Educated at Cambridge University and the University of London (Ph.D., nutrition, 1959). Served since 1983 as a senior adviser, with an emphasis on nutrition policy, iron- and iodine-deficiency disorders, vitamin A deficiency, and the protection, promotion, and support of breastfeeding. Served as UNICEF representative in Brasilia (1980–83), in New Delhi (1976–80), and with the Food and Agriculture Organization of the United Nations (FAO) in New Delhi supporting UNICEF programs (1972–76). Secretary of the British Nutrition Foundation (1971–72). Worked in FAO in Cairo (1969–70), supporting nutrition programs in the Middle East; and in the Nutrition Branch of the Ministry of Agriculture, Fisheries and Food, in London. Author of numerous monographs and articles, including: "Breast-Feeding and Growth Monitoring," with L. Hendrata, *International Journal of Gynecology and Obstetrics*, 31 (supplement 1990); "Nutrition Delivery System," *Indian Journal of Nutrition and Dietetics*, 16 (1979); "Role of Government," in *Nutrition in the Community*, ed. Donald S. McLaren (1976); "Nutrition Education—Education in Child Care," *Indian Pediatrics*, 10 (1973); and coauthor, with Bruce Johnston, *Manual on Food and Nutrition Policy* (1969). Born in Cardiff, United Kingdom, 1932. Address: Programme Division, UNICEF, UNICEF House, Three United Nations Plaza, New York, NY 10017.

Abraham Horwitz

Abraham Horwitz, director emeritus, Pan American Sanitary Bureau, Pan American Health Organization (PAHO), World Health Organization. President, Pan American Health and Education Foundation. Educated at the Universidad de Chile (M.D., with specialization in communicable diseases and public health) and the Johns Hopkins University. Chairman of the International Vitamin A Consultative Group, the UN Subcommittee on Nutrition, and the Advisory Group on Nutrition. Consultant to the director of PAHO. Chaired the committee on International Nutritional Programs of the National Research Council. As director of the Pan American Sanitary Bureau (1958–75), led in the creation of a Ten-Year Health Plan for the Americas, with a total investment reaching over $6.2 billion by 1977. A founder of the national health service in Chile, served as its assistant director. Former professor of bacteriology and immunology in the School of Medicine of the Universidad de Chile and director of its School of Public Health. Has written over three hundred articles in the fields of epidemiology, communicable diseases, preventive medicine, nutrition, and public health. Coeditor, *Nutrition in the Elderly* (1989), and author, *Infección Meningococcica en Chile* (1942). Honored by PAHO with the establishment of an annual Abraham Horwitz Award for Inter-

American Health. Recipient of numerous awards by governments in the Americas. Born in Santiago, Chile. Address: Pan American Health Organization, 525 Twenty-Third Street, N.W., Washington, DC 20037.

Norge W. Jerome

Norge W. Jerome, director, Office of Nutrition, Bureau of Science and Technology, U.S. Agency for International Development. Educated at Howard University and the University of Wisconsin at Madison (Ph.D., human nutrition, 1966). Director, Community Health Division, Department of Preventive Medicine, University of Kansas Medical Center; head, Community Nutrition Laboratory; and professor. Research and teaching areas include: nutrition and anthropological research techniques to determine patterns of food intake and dietary change; nutritional epidemiology; and international nutrition. Directs field research in the United States, the Caribbean, and in North Africa. Author of books and numerous journal articles, including: "Dietary Intake and Nutritional Status of Older U.S. Blacks: An Overview," in *Proceedings of the Conference on Aging Research on Black Populations* (in press); "Dietary Patterning and Change: A Continuous Process," *Contemporary Nutrition*, 7, no. 6 (1982); coauthor, with J. G. McCleery and I. D. Wolf, *Help Yourself* (1981); with R. Kandel and G. Pelto, *Nutritional Anthropology: Contemporary Approaches to Diet and Culture* (1980); and "Changing Nutritional Styles within the Context of the Modern Family," in *Family Health Care*, vol. 1 (1979). Associate editor, *Journal of Nutrition Education*. Born in Grenada, West Indies. Address: Office of Nutrition, Agency for International Development, 411B-SA 18, Department of State, Washington, DC 20523.

Liu Dong-sheng

Liu Dong-sheng, professor of nutrition, Institute of Nutrition and Food Hygiene, Chinese Academy of Preventive Medicine. Educated at West China Union University in Cheng-Duo and the Beijing Union Medical College. Research associate, Chinese Academy of Medical Sciences (1957–82) and at the National Institute of Hygiene. Dietician at the Chinese American Hospital in Shanghai. Consulting editor, *Chinese Journal of Pediatrics*. Food consultant to the Beijing Municipal Government. Vice-president of the Maternal and Child Nutrition Association and of the Chinese Child Food Science Society. Editor, *Problems in Home Nutrition* (1984) and *Studies on Infant Milk Substitutes in Rural Areas* (1979). Author, *Infant Feeding Practice* (1980). Has written numerous journal articles, including: "Studies on Iron-Deficiency Anemia of Preschool Children: Therapeutic Effect of Iron, Ascorbic Acid, and Iron-fortified Soft Drink Powder in the Treatment of Iron-Deficiency Anemia," *Acta Nutrimenta Sinica*, 5, no. 1 (1983); "The Effect of

Different Levels of Dietary Protein on the Growth and Nitrogen Metabolism of Two- and Three-Year-Old Children," *Journal of the Institute of Health*, 9, no. 3 (1980); and "Preparation and Nutritive Value of a Milk Substitute," *Chinese Medical Journal*, 92, no. 2 (1979). Honored for research on and development of food standards for infants and children, and the prevention of iron-deficiency anemia among preschool children. Born in Hunan Province, China, 1925. Address: Institute of Nutrition and Food Hygiene, Chinese Academy of Preventive Medicine, 29 Nan Wei Road, Beijing 100050, China.

Tshire O. Maribe

Tshire O. Maribe, chief nutritionist, Ministry of Health, Republic of Botswana. Educated at the University College of Sierra Leone (B.Sc., home economics, 1976) and the University of Kentucky (M.Sc., food science and nutrition, 1981). Also studied at the University College of Botswana, Lesotho, and Swaziland; Cornell University; and in Ghana. Has served in numerous positions, as a nutrition planner, in human resource planning, financial and budgetary management, and in community development. Research focus on the growth monitoring of children and nutritional surveillance systems. Coordinator of the thirteen-nation East, Central, and Southern Africa Food and Nutrition Cooperation organization. Helped develop and is a member of the committee monitoring the national food strategy in Botswana. Serves on the drought management committee that developed an early warning system. Has presented papers at international meetings and has authored reports, including: "Drought Relief Planning and Management," presented at the Third African Congress on Food and Nutrition, in Zimbabwe (1988); "The Practice of National Health Institute Post-Basic Community Health Nurses: Evaluation Research" (1985); "Growth Monitoring Experiences in Botswana," presented at a UNICEF conference in New York (1985); and "Update on the Nutrition Surveillance System in Botswana," presented at a conference in Kenya (1982). Address: Family Health Division, Ministry of Health, P. O. Box 992, Gaborone, Botswana.

Judith S. McGuire

Judith S. McGuire, nutritionist, Population, Health, and Nutrition Division, the World Bank. Educated at Wellesley College and the Massachusetts Institute of Technology (Ph.D., nutritional biochemistry and metabolism, 1979). Resident fellow at Resources for the Future (1985–88). Nutrition policy advisor at the U.S. Agency for International Development (1981–85). Nutrition analyst at the Food and Nutrition Service, U.S. Department of Agriculture. Received an International Affairs Fellowship from the Council on Foreign Relations. Worked in Kenya as a nutrition policy advisor (1980) and in Guatemala as principal investigator for a study on "Seasonality of Energy Expenditure in Rural Guatemalan Women" (1977–79). Research areas include: nutrition policy, essential micronutrient deficiencies, and women's nutrition. Coauthor with B. M. Popkin, *Helping Women Improve Nutrition in the Developing World: Beating the Zero Sum Game,* World Bank Technical Paper no. 114 (1990); with E. Kennedy, *Successful Nutrition Programs in Africa—What Makes Them Work* (1990); with O. Abosede, *Improving Women's and Children's Nutrition in Africa,* a World Bank Issues Paper (1989); with J. E. Austin, *Beyond Survival: Children's Growth for National Development,* a UNICEF Report (1987). Born in Montclair, New Jersey, 1950. Address: Population, Health and Nutrition Division, Population and Human Resources Department, The World Bank, 1818 H Street, N.W., Washington, DC 20433.

Fernando Monckeberg B.

Fernando Monckeberg B., founder and director, Instituto de Nutrición y Tecnología de los Alimentos, Universidad de Chile. President of the Chilean Nutrition Foundation and the Latin American Society of Nutrition. Founder of the Foundation of Infantile Nutrition (CONIN) and of the Latin American Society of Pediatric Research. Educated at the Patrocinio de San Jose and in medicine at the Universidad de Chile. Principal research areas include: the effects of malnutrition and sensory deprivation on child development, metabolic alterations, and central nervous system development. Oversees the treatment of undernourished children at CONIN, which includes thirty-three recovery centers and twelve hundred pediatric beds. Founder and president of the Foundation for Adoption. Directed the university's Laboratory of Pediatric Research, and professor of pediatrics and of nutrition. Author of nearly two hundred articles and monographs, and author and editor of books, including: *Desnutrición Infantil: Fisiopatologia, Clinica, Tratamiento y Prevención, Nuestra Experiencia y Contribución* (1988); *Checkmate to Underdevelopment* (1975); and "The Effect of Malnutrition on Physical Growth and Brain Development," in *Brain Function and Malnutrition: Neuropsychological Methods of Assessment,* ed. J. W. Prescott, et. al. (1975). Recipient of numerous honors, including the Abraham Horwitz Prize of the Pan American Health Education Foundation and the Christopherson Prize of the American Academy of Pediatrics. Born in Santiago, Chile, 1920. Address: Instituto de Nutrición y Tecnología de los Alimentos, Universidad de Chile, Casilla 138-11, Santiago, Chile.

John S. Niederhauser

John S. Niederhauser, cofounder, Centro Internacional de la Papa (International Potato Center), Peru, and former director, Mexican Potato Improvement Project and Inter-American Potato Program. Educated at Cornell University (Ph.D., 1943).

Held several posts at the Rockefeller Foundation: as plant pathologist in Mexico; director, International Potato Program; and as associate director of agricultural science. Founder of the Programa Regional Cooperativo de Papa (PRECODEPA), a new model and strategy for regional cooperation in agricultural research and production. Held several university teaching and research positions, at Cornell University, the Max Planck Institute in West Germany, and at the University of Arizona. His research has been devoted to the control of potato late blight and to the breeding of a durable resistance. He pioneered the concept of "horizontal resistance," which led to the development of new potato varieties. His work as a consultant to Polish potato farmers led to the establishment in Mexico in 1990 of the International Cooperative Potato Late Blight Project. Recipient of the Medal of Merit, awarded by Mexico's Ministry of Agriculture (1981), and the Premio Mexico de Fitopatologia, of the Mexico Phytopathological Society (1985). Born in Seattle, Washington, 1916. Address: 2474 Camino Valle Verde, Tucson, AZ 85715.

V. Rahmathullah

V. Rahmathullah, director, Child Development Unit, Aravind Children's Hospital. Educated at the Lady Hardings Medical College, Delhi University (M.B.B.S. degree, 1957), and at the London School of Hygiene and Tropical Medicine, University of London (Ross Institute Scholar; Diploma in tropical public health, 1976). Former director, Aravind Children's Hospital. A physician and surgeon at several hospitals. Lectured and trained interns at St. John's Medical College in Bangalore. Medical adviser to the United Planter's Association of Southern India, with responsibility for maternal and child health in a community of two hundred fifty thousand persons, and the development of the Link Worker program, a national model of primary health care. Author of numerous papers, including: "Alternative Approaches to Perinatal and Neonatal Care in Rural Communities," *Indian Pediatric Journal* (1989); "Link Workers: A Success Story on Raising Health Consciousness among Plantation Workers," *Proceedings* of the Third International Conference of the World Public Health Association (1981); "Trends in Births and Deaths in South Indian Plantations," *Tropical Doctor* (October 1981); and "A Double Blind Study on Anemia and Productivity," *Nutritional Society of India* (1979). Past president of the Indian Medical Association. Member of the All India Council of the Family Planning Association and the Task Force on Vitamin A. Fellow of the Royal Society of Tropical Medicine and Hygiene, London. Born in Basra, Iraq, 1930. Address: Child Development Unit, Aravind Children's Hospital, 28, Kamarajar Street, Madurai 625 020, India.

Eduardo L. Roberto

Eduardo L. Roberto, Coca-Cola Foundation Professor of International Marketing, Asian Institute of Management. Educated at De LaSalle University in Manila and

Northwestern University (M.S., behavioral science; Ph.D., marketing, 1973). A consultant to governments and corporations in southeast Asia, and to international organizations in the fields of social and population research, marketing, and management planning and research. President and chairman, ER Associates, Inc., a survey research and training firm. Former executive vice-president of Consumer Pulse, Inc., the largest survey research organization in southeast Asia. Program director for contraceptive social marketing, Population Center Foundation; and executive director, International Council on the Management of Population Programmes. Coauthor, with Philip Kotler, *Social Marketing: Strategies for Changing Public Behavior* (1989); author, *Applied Marketing Research* (1987); "Skills for Management Development in Population Programs," in *Management Development in Population Programs,* ed. S. C. Jain, et. al. (1981); and *Strategic Decision Making in a Social Program: The Case of Family Planning Diffusion* (1975); along with numerous journal articles. Served as president of the Marketing and Opinion Research Society of the Philippines and as director of the Philippine Board of Advertising. Recipient of the Philippine Marketing Association AGORA Award for achievement in marketing education. Born in Bataan, The Philippines. Address: Asian Institute of Management, 123 Paseo de Roxas, P. O. Box 898, Makati, Metro Manila, The Philippines.

Barbara A. Underwood

Barbara A. Underwood, assistant director for International Program Activities, National Eye Institute, National Institutes of Health. Educated at the University of California at Santa Barbara, Cornell University, and Columbia University (Ph.D., nutritional biochemistry, 1962). Lecturer, Department of International Health, The Johns Hopkins University. Former professor of nutrition at the University of Maryland School of Medicine; Institute of Human Nutrition, Columbia University; director of the Division of Biological Health, Pennsylvania State University; resident coordinator, United Nations University Food and Nutrition Program; and associate professor, Massachusetts Institute of Technology. Consultant on nutrition education and training, infant and child-feeding practices, and vitamin A deficiency. Author and editor of more than one hundred publications, including: "Blinding Malnutrition: A Preventable Scourge," in *Nutritional Problems of Children in the Developing World* (forthcoming); "Vitamin A Deficiency in Pregnancy, Lactation, and the Nursing Child," with J. C. Wallingford, in *Vitamin A Deficiency and Its Control* (1986); "Relation of Serum Vitamins A and E and Carotenoid to the Risk of Cancer," with W. C. Willett, et. al., *New England Journal of Medicine* (1984); and *Nutrition Intervention Strategies in National Development* (1983). Vice president, International Union of Nutrition Sciences. Member of the UN Secretary's Group on Control of Vitamin A Deficiency. Born in Santa Ana, California, 1934. Address: National Eye Institute, Bldg. 31, Rm. 6A-17, NIH, 9000 Rockville Pike, Bethesda, MD 20892.

David L. Yeung

David L. Yeung, corporate nutrition coordinator, H. J. Heinz Company of Canada, Ltd. Educated at the University of Toronto (Ph.D., 1970). Associate professor of nutritional sciences, Faculty of Medicine, University of Toronto. Visiting professor, Sun Yat Sen University of Medical Sciences, Guangzhou, People's Republic of China (PRC), and honorary professor in the School of Public Health of West China University of Medical Sciences in Chengdu, PRC. Head, Heinz Institutes of Nutritional Sciences in Guangzhou, PRC, and at Mahidol University, Bangkok, Thailand. Chair, Infant Nutrition Institute. Nutrition consultant to the Beijing Pediatric Research Institute, Beijing Children's Hospital. Served as coordinator of the Nutrition Sciences Committee, Institute for the Study and Application of Integrated Development, Toronto, Canada. Member, Canadian Science Committee on Food and Nutrition; and consultant to the Canadian Paediatric Society. Former chairman, Geriatric Nutrition Committee, National Institute of Nutrition. Editor, *Heinz Nutritional Data*, 7th edition, (1990) and *Essays on Pediatric Nutrition* (1981). General editor, *Issues in Infant Nutrition: Practical Approaches for the Physician and Parents* (1989). Author, *Infant Nutrition: A Study of Feeding and Growth from Birth to Eighteen Months* (1983), and of over fifty journal articles. Has organized numerous international meetings in the fields of maternal and infant nutrition. Born in Hong Kong, 1939. Address: H. J. Heinz Company of Canada, Ltd., North American Life Centre, 5650 Yonge Street, 16th Floor, North Fork, Ontario M2M 4G3, Canada.

About the Editor and the Sponsors

Neil G. Kotler is a program specialist in the Office of Interdisciplinary Studies, Smithsonian Institution. He studied at Brandeis University and The University of Chicago, where he received his Ph.D. in political science. For ten years he was a legislative assistant in the U.S. House of Representatives and was a staff member of the Subcommittee on the City, the House Banking Committee. He has written and edited articles and books, including *The History of Eritrea* (Addis Ababa, Ethiopia: Ministry of Education, 1966) which was an outgrowth of his service as a Peace Corps volunteer in Asmara, Ethiopia. He is editor of *Sharing Innovation: Global Perspectives on Food, Agriculture, and Rural Development* (Smithsonian Institution Press, 1990), coeditor of *Completing the Food Chain: Strategies for Combating Hunger and Malnutrition* (Smithsonian Institution Press, 1989), and an editor of *Social Marketing: Strategies for Changing Public Behavior,* authored by Philip Kotler and Eduardo L. Roberto (Free Press/Macmillan, 1989).

The International Life Sciences Institute-North America

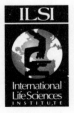

The International Life Sciences Institute (ILSI) is a nonprofit, worldwide foundation established in 1978 to advance the understanding of scientific issues relating to nutrition, food safety, toxicology, and the environment and to promote regulatory harmonization in these areas. By bringing together scientists from academia, government, and industry, ILSI seeks a balanced approach to solving problems with broad implications for the well-being of the general public. ILSI's standards, the quality of the research it supports, and the worldwide as well as regional meetings it sponsors are recognized by the scientific community throughout the world. ILSI is affiliated with the World Health Organization as a nongovernmental organization and has specialized consultative status with the Food and Agriculture Organization of the United Nations. Headquartered in Washington, D.C., ILSI has branches in Argentina, Australia, Brazil, Europe, Japan, Mexico, and North America, with branches under consideration elsewhere.

The International Rice Research Institute

IRRI One out of every three persons on earth depends on rice for more than half of his or her daily food. The International Rice Research Institute (IRRI) in Los Baños, the Philippines, is an autonomous, nonprofit agricultural research and training center whose goals are to alleviate hunger and malnourishment by applying science to agriculture and enabling resource-poor farmers to produce more rice from limited land. IRRI conducts research to increase total food production in rice-based farming systems. In the 1960s IRRI became the laboratory for developing high-yielding rice varieties that generated the Green Revolution in Asia.

Most of IRRI's research is undertaken in cooperation with national agricultural development programs and universities. Today, about six thousand IRRI-trained scientists and rice specialists work as members of national rice research and development teams in Asia, Africa, and Latin America.

IRRI is one of thirteen nonprofit international research and training centers supported by the Consultative Group on International Agricultural Research (CGIAR), a consortium of fifty donor nations, international and regional organizations, and private foundations, sponsored by the Food and Agriculture Organization of the United Nations, the World Bank, and the United Nations Development Programme.